PAINFUL QUESTIONS...

- Do you have constant pain in your neck, back, or shoulders that won't go away?

- Have you tried conventional and alternative treatments like herbs and acupuncture, but your problems still persist?

- Do you suffer from new, sometimes disabling conditions, such as carpal tunnel syndrome, fibromyalgia, and post-polio syndrome—all part of tension myositis syndrome—and wonder if they can be treated?

- Do your efforts to cure your chronic pain or illness seem like a Sisyphean endeavor?

- Are you fearful or suspicious of expensive medical procedures involving drugs and surgery that might fail to alleviate your condition?

- Do you want to understand how your mind and body can interact to solve your pain problems?

If your answers are "yes," don't despair. Fighting pain is not a losing cause. Pioneering physician Dr. John E. Sarno, who has helped thousands of relieved patients, introduces your most powerful weapon in the war on pain and disability...

THE MINDBODY PRESCRIPTION

The Mindbody Prescription

Healing the Body,
Healing the Pain

John E. Sarno, M.D.

GRAND CENTRAL
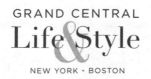
Life & Style
NEW YORK · BOSTON

Grand Central Life & Style
Hachette Book Group
1290 Avenue of the Americas
New York, NY 10104

www.HachetteBookGroup.com

Printed in the United States of America

Originally published in hardcover by Hachette Book Group.

First Trade Edition: October 1999
20 19

Grand Central Life & Style is an imprint of Grand Central Publishing.
The Grand Central Life & Style name and logo are trademarks of Hachette Book Group, Inc.

The publisher is not responsible for websites (or their content) that are not owned by the publisher.

The Library of Congress has cataloged the hardcover edition as follows:

Sarno, John E.
    The mindbody prescription : healing the body, healing the pain / John E. Sarno.
        p.   cm.
    Includes index.
    ISBN 0-446-52076-4
    1. Medicine, Psychosomatic.   2. Pain—Psychosomatic aspects.
3. Mind and body therapies.   I. Title.
RC49.S34   1998
616'.0472—dc21   97-41031
                                                          CIP

ISBN 978-0446-67515-4 (pbk.)

Dedicated with gratitude and
affection to my patients:
the source of my knowledge
and the fount of my pleasure in
the practice of medicine.

Acknowledgments

I am indebted to these busy people who were kind enough to read and critique parts or all of the text: Frances Anderson, Jim Campobello, Stanley Coen, Arlene Feinblatt, Marion Hart, Ruth Imber, Ira Rashbaum and Eric Sherman. I am additionally grateful to the psychotherapists in this group who have worked with me through the years and contributed immensely to my understanding of the psychodynamics of the unconscious.

As a result of her illustrious career as medical author and editor, the suggestions of my wife, Martha Taylor Sarno, were extremely valuable.

I have been particularly fortunate in having found a sensitive, diplomatic and very effective literary agent in Alice Martell. Publication bumps were minimal, but she was most helpful in smoothing the few there were.

The editor of *Healing Back Pain* and original editor of this book was Susan Suffes, who was a joy to work with; along the way she decided on a career change and left Warner Books. However, fortune smiled on me once more when Susan Sandler became my editor. Susan is from the old school—she edits. I am most grateful for her stylistic and organizational changes and embarrassed by what some of the text would have looked like without her editing.

And finally, literally and figuratively, there is Mary Oland, my secretary, indefatigable typist and conqueror of the computer. I have marveled at her good humor in the face of innumerable changes and copies. Thank you, Mary.

Contents

Preface

Pain, disability, misinformation, fear—that quartet has plagued the Western world for decades and the plague shows no sign of abating. Back, neck and limb pain are rampant, and statistics indicate that the epidemic is spreading. Disability in American industry from low back pain continues to increase year by year.

Industries that employ large numbers of people working at computers are experiencing great disability and health insurance problems because of a new pain disorder known as *repetitive stress injury* (RSI). Millions of Americans, mostly women, suffer from a painful malady of unknown cause called fibromyalgia. While gigantic medical industries have arisen to diagnose and treat these conditions, the plague continues.

This book is about that epidemic. It describes both a clinical experience that has identified the cause of the pain disorders and a method of treating them. Sadly, mainstream medicine rejects the diagnosis because it is based on the theory that the physical symptoms are initiated by emotional phenomena. Intelligent laymen in large numbers have embraced the concept, however, no doubt because they are not burdened by the bias imposed by a traditional medical education.

As if the pain epidemic were not of sufficient magnitude, a large group of physical disorders have been identified as *equivalents* of the pain syndrome, since they appear to stem from the same psychological process. These maladies have occurred commonly for years and, taken together with the widespread pain maladies, are universal in Western society. I refer to many of the headaches, gastrointestinal symptoms and allergies, as well as respiratory, dermatologic, genitourinary and gynecologic conditions that are the stuff of everyday life.

If most of these are psychogenic—that is, they originate in the mind (and it is my goal to demonstrate that they are)—we have a public health problem of staggering proportions. The medical, humanitarian and economic implications are obvious and will be enumerated.

This book is about emotions, illness and wellness, how they are related and what one can do to enhance good health and combat certain physical conditions. The ideas are based on twenty-four years of successfully treating an emotionally induced physical disorder known as the Tension Myositis Syndrome (TMS). Although I will provide an up-to-date description of that condition, my major focus is the impact of the emotions on bodily function.

That connection came close to being accepted by Western medicine in the first half of the twentieth century and then fell into almost total disrepute. Repudiation of psychoanalytic theory, increased interest in laboratory research and the tendency of doctors to shy away from psychological matters (they see themselves as engineers to the human body) are the likely reasons for this historical trend. As the century draws to a close, few practitioners, either in physical or psychological medicine, believe that unconscious, repressed emotions initiate physical illness. Psychoanalysts are the only clinicians who have held to that concept, but their influence in the larger fields of psychiatry and general medicine is limited. In the physical medicine specialties virtually no one adheres to the idea.

Despite the lack of interest of mainstream medicine, much has been written on the "mind-body connection." Careful studies have been conducted that relate psychological factors to pathological conditions such as coronary artery disease and hypertension. I know of only one investigator out-side the field of psychoanalysis who has identified uncon-scious emotions as the cause of a physical illness. One reads of stress, anger, anxiety, loneliness, depression, but they are dis-cussed as conscious, perceived emotions. In many instances these feelings are thought to aggravate underlying structural pathological processes, such as herniated discs, fibromyalgia or repetitive stress injury.

In view of the widespread Freud-bashing of recent years I may be courting disapproval to state that my concepts de-scend from Freud's clinical observations and theories. But I know this only in retrospect, for I did not set out to prove Freud right. My developing ideas were the consequence of clinical observations; they were not based on preconceived notions about the mindbody connection. As with Freud's pa-tients, I found that my patients' physical symptoms were the direct result of strong feelings repressed in the unconscious. In addition, I have drawn on the concepts of three other psy-choanalysts: Franz Alexander, founder of the Chicago Insti-tute for Psychoanalysis, did pioneer work in mindbody medicine in this century; Heinz Kohut conceptualized what is known as Self Psychology and pointed out the importance of narcissistic rage; Stanley Coen suggested the crucial idea that the mindbody disorder I was studying (TMS) was a de-fense, an avoidance strategy designed to turn attention away from frightening repressed feelings.

This book addresses physical disorders that are caused by repressed, unconscious feelings. Because these disorders are very specific, they can be accurately diagnosed and success-fully treated.

The Tension Myositis Syndrome is currently the most common emotionally induced disorder in the United States, and probably in the Western world. Since the publication of *Healing Back Pain*, other painful conditions of significant public health importance have emerged. They, too, are manifestations of TMS.

The book is laid out in three parts. Part I is a discussion of the psychology that induces these physical maladies, and it includes a chapter that might be called a bridge, for it describes the psychoneurophysiology of psychogenic processes: in other words, how emotions stimulate the brain to produce physical symptoms. After traversing this bridge (which sounds more formidable than it is), Part II takes up the various emotionally induced physical maladies, beginning with TMS, the disorder that introduced me to the world of mindbody medicine, and including such ailments as the common disturbances of the gastrointestinal tract, headaches, allergies and skin disorders.

Part III discusses treatment for these disorders.

For those who are interested, an appendix covers the more academic aspects of the mindbody (psychosomatic) process.

A word of caution to the reader: What follows is a description of my clinical experience and the theories derived from my work. No one should assume that his or her symptoms are psychologically caused until a physician has ruled out the possibility of serious disease.

Introduction: A Historical Perspective

Like a wildly growing cancer, the problem of pain of all kinds has become, since my graduation from medical school, a major epidemic in most of the industrialized countries of the Western world. The diagnosis and treatment of these disorders in the United States is now a gargantuan industry. The back pain problem alone costs the nation upward of seventy billion dollars a year, and if we add all the modern pain epidemics, such as carpal tunnel syndrome, the figure is probably twice that. One does not hear these medical problems described as epidemics, probably because they are not usually life-threatening, nor is the public fully aware of their financial, social and emotional ravages. That they do not threaten life is the only positive thing that can be said about them, since they can be more physically and emotionally disabling than many seemingly catastrophic disorders. A well-rehabilitated person with paralysis of both legs can lead an essentially normal life, while someone with severe chronic pain may be almost totally disabled, unable to work and capable of very little physical activity.

The immediate and inevitable question is, Why and how did this happen? After millions of years of evolution, have we suddenly become incapable of functioning normally? Are there architectural inadequacies in our bodies that have only become apparent in the last forty years? If these pain disorders are not caused by structural abnormalities, how else can these epidemics be explained?

My early work in the diagnosis and treatment of back, neck and shoulder pain syndromes was decidedly unpleasant and frustrating. The conventional diagnoses and conservative (nonsurgical) treatment methods yielded disappointing and inconsistent results. Even as I explained the rationales for diagnosis and treatment to patients, I was uncomfortable, for the explanations seemed to lack physiologic and anatomic logic. As far back as 1904 doctors had described a painful disorder of the muscles—variously called fibromyalgia, myofasciitis, fibrositis, fibromyositis—but no one had been able to identify the exact pathology or cause of the condition. Eventually I began to approach patients as though nothing were known about the cause of back pain. I soon realized the primary tissue involved was muscle. Something was happening to the muscles of the neck, shoulders, back and buttocks.

Because they are easily identified on X ray, most practitioners attributed the pain to a variety of structural abnormalities of the spine, such as normal aging changes, congenital abnormalities or malalignment. Others believed that the muscles were painful because they were weak, sprained or strained. Furthermore, back, neck or shoulder pain was often accompanied by pain and other neurological symptoms in an arm or leg. If, therefore, a structural abnormality was found in the vicinity of a spinal nerve whose destination was an arm or leg, the clinician would be strongly inclined to attribute the symptoms to that abnormality without concern for the rigors of a scientific diagnosis. However, a careful history and physical examination often revealed that the presumed culprit was innocent, that the bone or disc distortion could not account for the findings. Nevertheless, pain was still blamed on the spine.

An unlikely alliance arose among disparate disciplines. Chiropractors, for years roundly criticized by physicians as unscientific, slowly came to be fully accepted into the fraternity of diagnosers and treaters of the back. They had always maintained that structural abnormalities of the spine were the cause of back pain. Since doctors believed the same thing, it was inevitable that chiropractors would become members of the back therapy community. Other members of this therapeutic community are osteopaths, physiatrists (specialists in physical medicine and rehabilitation), orthopedists, neurologists, neurosurgeons, physical therapists, acupuncturists, kinesiologists and a host of others who use special regimens of exercise or massage. What they have in common is the idea that the spine and/or its surrounding musculature is deficient, easily injured and in need of some kind of physical intervention. Surgery is the most drastic and one of the most common.

Because some sort of structurally induced inflammation, *whose nature has never been elucidated*, is said to be responsible for much of the pain, large numbers of nonsteroidal and steroidal medications are prescribed.

In view of the many diagnostic and therapeutic programs now used in the management of these pain syndromes, any significant disruption in the application of existing therapies would create financial havoc, for the diagnosis and treatment of chronic pain is now a gigantic industry in the United States. But accurate diagnosis and treatment would save enormous amounts of money.

In the early 1970s, in the midst of this burgeoning epidemic, I began to doubt the validity of the conventional diagnoses, and therefore treatment, of the syndromes of neck, shoulder and back pain. A closer look had suggested that back muscles, from the back of the head to the buttocks, were the primary tissues involved. This confirmed the work of all those through the years who described what they called fibromyalgia, fibrositis or myofascial pain. My study of the literature and growing experience with patients suggested that those maladies were part of a pain disorder I call the Tension Myositis Syndrome (TMS). (*Myositis* means physiologic alteration of muscles.) TMS is a painful but harmless change of state in muscles.

But what of the neurological signs and symptoms in the legs and arms? For a while I thought they must be caused by structural compression in the spine or that mysterious "inflammation" so often cited by other practitioners. As the number of inconsistencies mounted, however, I was forced to the conclusion that the process causing the muscle pain was responsible for the nerve symptoms as well. But what was that process?

When physicians take a patient's history they routinely inquire about past or current medical disorders or symptoms. I found that 88 percent of my pain patients had a history of minor gastrointestinal maladies such as heartburn, pre-ulcer symptoms, hiatus hernia, colitis, spastic colon, irritable bowel syndrome and other tension-induced reactions like tension headache, migraine headache, eczema and frequent urination. Although not all practitioners agree that these disorders are related to psychological or emotional phenomena, my clinical experience as a family physician and my own personal medical history made me quite comfortable with that conclusion. For example, for a number of years I had experienced regular migraine headaches, complete with typical visual "lights" prior to the onset of headache. Someone suggested that repressed anger might be the basis for them. The next time I had the "lights"—harbinger of a headache—I sat down and tried to think of what anger I might be repressing. I failed to find an answer, *but for the first time in my life I didn't get a headache.* It was powerful evidence that migraine headache was caused by emotional phenomena.

It was, therefore, logical to hypothesize that these back muscle pains might fall into the same group of emotionally induced physical disorders. When I put the idea to the test, by telling patients that I thought their pain was the result of "tension," I was astonished to observe that those who accepted the diagnosis got better. Those who rejected it remained unchanged.

In those early days all my patients had physical therapy administered by therapists whom I had briefed to inform patients that the therapy was designed to provide temporary relief from symptoms, but that real recovery depended on recognizing the nature of the process. Those who improved agreed with the diagnosis. This was similar to my experience with migraine: Acknowledgment of an emotional role in the genesis of symptoms somehow banished those symptoms. Many years would pass before I understood the reason for this fascinating, mysterious phenomenon.

At the time, telling patients that I thought their pain was caused by "tension" was difficult. Any physician would scoff at this idea; the average person would be insulted if you suggested that some physical symptom was "in the head." That was a phrase I avoided assiduously because of its pejorative connotation, although the patient often introduced it. Sometimes I was able to explain the connection between tension and pain satisfactorily, but I was quite handicapped because of my own poor understanding of the psychodynamics involved. Instead I talked about certain personality characteristics that appeared to be common in people with TMS and how these characteristics might lead to tension and anxiety. I suggested that the symptoms were a physical rather than emotional expression of anxiety and that people who were hardworking, conscientious, responsible, compulsive and perfectionistic were prone to TMS. I could not provide a clinical definition of the word *tension* but it was a word with which people could identify. *Psychological* and *emotional* were bad words that implied there was something strange about you; I avoided the word *psychosomatic* because to most people it meant the pain was phony or imaginary. Nevertheless, I continued to make the diagnosis, and my rate of success in treatment began to rise substantially. I now felt I understood the nature of the disorder and could predict with some accuracy who would get better and who wouldn't.

On physical examination almost every patient was found to have tenderness on palpation of (pressing on) certain muscles regardless of where in the neck or back they felt pain. For example, someone might have pain only in the right lower back but on examination felt pain when I pressed on the top of both shoulders (upper trapezius muscles), the small of the back on both sides (lumbar paraspinal muscles), and the outer part of both buttocks (gluteal muscles). This consistent finding strongly suggested that the syndrome originated in the central nervous system (brain) rather than in a local structural abnormality.

By the mid-1970s I had concluded that the majority of neck, shoulder and back pain syndromes, along with the associated pain often seen in the legs and arms, was the result of a psychologically induced process, which made it a classical psychosomatic condition. That is, emotional factors were setting off a reaction in certain tissues in the body that resulted in pain and other neurologic symptoms.

What was the nature of this reaction? The physical therapy treatment consisted of deep heat (delivered as high-frequency sound waves), deep massage and active exercise of the involved muscles. Most patients reported at least temporary relief. Since I knew that these treatment modalities increased the local circulation of blood, it was logical to conclude that the cause of the symptoms was a reduction in blood flow to the involved tissues. The circulation of blood is under the control of a subsystem of the central nervous system known as the autonomic nervous system. Many of the other mindbody disorders (peptic ulcer, colitis, migraine and tension headache) are also mediated through the autonomic system. Nothing could be simpler: Something in the brain decides to initiate this process; autonomic centers are activated, and within milliseconds the circulation to the involved areas is reduced. This means that these tissues are now deprived of their full complement of oxygen, which is almost certainly the reason for the symptoms. This correlated with the finding of two German investigators in 1975 that there was evidence of mild oxygen deprivation in the nuclei of muscle cells of patients with back pain, as well as with studies reported in the medical literature by a team of Swedish rheumatologists in the 1980s.

Since it provided a logical explanation for the symptoms, I proceeded on the premise that oxygen deprivation causes pain. Further, even if the cause of the pain should prove to be some other brain-induced process, it was still apparent that definitive treatment had to be directed at the brain, not the local tissues.

I told my patients there was really nothing wrong with their backs. I explained that they had a harmless condition that must be treated through the mind, not the body. Awareness, insight, knowledge and information were the magic medicines that would cure this disorder—and nothing else could do it.

In 1979 I instituted the practice of bringing patients together and lecturing them on the physical and psychological details of TMS. The logic was clear: If information was the cure, I ought to be doing a better job of providing it. These lectures now represent the cornerstone of the therapeutic program and appear to be all that is necessary for 80 to 90 percent of those who go on to complete recovery.

My view of the problem in the early 1980s is best illustrated by a letter I wrote to *New York Times* columnist Russell Baker, whose August 16, 1981, column was titled "Where Have All the Ulcers Gone?" Since I suspected it would be of interest to him, on September 23, 1981, I sent the following letter:

Dear Mr. Baker:

Because you are a well-informed man, I thought you would be interested in knowing the real reason for the decline in the incidence of ulcers, about which you wrote awhile back. Gastric and duodenal ulcers are members of a family of physical disorders which, as you correctly reported, reflect the presence of large quantities of tension. Other members of this villainous family are colitis, spastic colon, tension headache and garden variety allergies, to name some of the most prominent. There is another one, however, which has escaped the notice of the medical community, or rather survived in the guise of being something else, and it is a very important one for it has assumed the role of the previously ubiquitous ulcer. Why this switch should have occurred is a very interesting story, to which I shall return in a moment. This other disorder is none other than the common backache (or neck or shoulder ache). For years it has been assumed that back pain is due to some deficiency of the spine and related structures, but this is merely a diagnostic smoke screen which has successfully obfuscated doctors and other practitioners. In fact, back pain is due to hyperactivity in that same branch of the nervous system which causes ulcers, the stimulus for which is the same old bugaboo, tension.

I am very serious in this assertion and have published my views in the medical literature. However, a certain degree of light-heartedness is appropriate since even the most painful and disabling of these is still reflective of a very benign process—much more so than ulcers which can bleed or perforate and become rather messy. All of these disorders are members of the same family and represent variants of a similar underlying process, i.e., tension producing physical manifestations, the definition of a psychosomatic disorder. Heart attacks are manifestations of a more serious kind of psychosomatic process and not equatable with peptic ulcer.

Now to the question of why the switch. This is not comprehensible unless one realizes that the purpose of a physical manifestation of tension is to deceive. Our brains have decided that *feeling tense*, which is the appropriate response to *being tense*, is too unpleasant to bear and is not as socially acceptable as having something "physically" wrong. And so the brain makes a few adjustments in circuitry and instead of looking and acting like a nervous wreck, presto—a bellyache or a backache. The reason why the ulcer had to go was that everybody began to realize that it was a phony, that it really meant tension, and that's not socially acceptable.

The old backache has always been what it is now, a tension equivalent, but nobody paid much attention to it until the advent of modern medicine. Here, said the brain, is a natural. Everybody thinks backaches are the last word in a "physical" disorder and so it's a perfect substitute for tension. The ulcer has lost its value—up the backache as the new but thoroughly hidden standard bearer for the army of the tense.

And so it is that practically everyone you talk to has a backache story to tell. The incidence of all kinds of pain syndromes involving the backside of western *Homo sapiens* has risen dramatically in the last twenty years or so, while the discredited ulcer is fading into obscurity.

Isn't that a fascinating story?

A few days later I received the following note, reprinted with Mr. Baker's kind permission:

Dear Dr. Sarno:

That's a fascinating story indeed and casts some light on my own "backache." This affliction comes over me after four or five hours at the typewriter when I am performing, as it were, for an audience. It is often particularly bad when I am aware the writing is going badly.

Last week I had occasion to help my son move and warned him that I'd probably have to drop out after a few hours on account of my back. The moving, in fact, was rather enjoyable, at least in the sense that it was mindless labor, fetching, lifting and hauling, performed in a pleasant rustic atmosphere with my mind thoroughly relaxed. After a ten-hour day at it, I remembered my back for the first time since morning, and then only to remark that it hadn't bothered me all day.

Yrs,

Russell Baker

In 1981, I believed that physical manifestations were a substitute for anxiety. Later, a change in concept led me to a much better understanding of the problem and, accordingly, greater effectiveness in treating it. The subtle but important shift was that unconscious emotional phenomena *necessitated* physical symptoms.

And, of course, ulcers have not faded into obscurity; they are now being attributed to the presence of a bacterium in the stomach. It is my opinion that they are still stress-induced and that the bacterium is merely part of the process. They are not as common as they used to be and do not occur as frequently as the pain disorders.

In 1982 I conducted the first follow-up survey of my patients. One hundred and seventy-seven patients whose charts were drawn randomly from those who had been treated between 1978 and 1981 were interviewed about their level of pain and their functional ability. Seventy-six percent were leading normal lives and were essentially free of pain. Fourteen patients were somewhat improved and twenty-eight (16 percent) were considered treatment failures.

Two important facts about this group of patients should be noted: Before coming to see me most of them had long histories of back pain and had received multiple treatments, including surgery for some, yet they still continued to have severe symptoms; also, I had not screened any of them before they made an appointment. Since 1987 I have interviewed patients calling for an appointment to determine whether they are appropriate for our program. Most of the large population of people with these pain syndromes reject the idea of an emotionally induced process and would, therefore, derive no benefit from our therapeutic program, since acceptance of the diagnosis is essential to a successful outcome. Currently I accept about 50 percent of those who call. When I am criticized for this selectivity I remind my critics that, like a surgeon who will not operate on a poor surgical risk, I am exercising my prerogative to work only with patients who have a reasonable chance for success. This selectivity is not only to my advantage; it spares the potential patient unnecessary expense and aggravation.

Despite this lack of selectivity prior to 1987, a second follow-up survey in 1987 revealed an increase in the effectiveness of the program since 1982. This time we made it more difficult for ourselves and limited the population surveyed to people with CT-scanned documented herniated discs. This abnormality is responsible for most back surgery, yet our experience shows that it is rarely responsible for the pain. One hundred and nine of these randomly selected patients were interviewed. One to three years after treatment, ninety-six (88 percent) were free of pain and leading normal lives, eleven people were somewhat better and only two were unchanged—a considerable improvement over the 1982 survey.

What was responsible for this significant improvement in our results? I had become more proficient at teaching the nature of TMS and was, therefore, more successful in stimulating confidence in the diagnosis; moreover, in 1985 I discontinued prescribing physical therapy. Although all the therapists were fully aware of the nature of the process they were treating and faithfully reinforced the concept that psychological and not physical factors were responsible for the pain, it became apparent that some patients would focus on the physical treatments, pay lip service to the ideas I was teaching, and have a placebo cure, if any (*placebo cure*—a cure based on blind faith and usually temporary). More subtly, by requiring physical treatment two or three times a week, we were focusing patients' attention on their bodies, whereas success in treatment depended on shifting concern from the physical to the emotional. The possible benefit of the physical therapy was heavily outweighed by its negative potential. I believe this played an important role in the improved statistics.

Although a third follow-up survey has not been done, I believe that our results are now even better than they were in 1987. I attribute this to the selectivity process as well as to a major leap in my understanding of the psychology of TMS.

While I was collaborating on a medical paper with a psychoanalyst colleague, Stanley Coen, he suggested that the physical symptoms were probably not a physical expression of anxiety, which had been my working hypothesis for many years, but were the result of what psychoanalysts call a defense mechanism, a term I find somewhat misleading in view of what it does. The purpose of a defense mechanism (in this case physical symptoms) is to divert people's attention to the body, so that they can *avoid* the awareness of or confrontation with certain unconscious (repressed) feelings. This new understanding of the role of repression was a major landmark in the journey upon which I had embarked roughly fifteen years before. Not only did this idea fit perfectly with the diagnosis, but for the first time I had an explanation of why people got better when they learned about and accepted what was going on. Now it was clear why someone in Peoria, Illinois, might read either of my books on TMS and make a complete recovery without ever having talked to or been examined by me. The mystery was solved. Once accepted by the patient, the knowledge of what was going on destroyed the brain's strategy. Although we had always known that TMS was a brain-induced process, we didn't know why the brain was doing it. Now it was clear that the symptoms were meant to draw the person's attention away from hidden emotions, and that by exposing the undercover operation and thereby ending it, the pain would disappear, as indeed it did.

While these ideas on the mindbody link represent the culmination of a twenty-four-year-long clinical experience, they are, in fact, the starting point for the body of this book. Though they developed out of my experience with the diagnosis and treatment of pain, I believe they have relevance to many medical conditions. Indeed, I believe that everyone has mindbody physical symptoms. Few people, if any, go through life without one or more such manifestations, for they reflect the evolutionary contemporary organization of the human psyche. Most importantly, these manifestations demonstrate that there is no separation between mind and body; that the two are inextricably intertwined. One cannot study the pathology of human disease without factoring in the role of the psyche. My experience with the common pain syndromes has demonstrated the folly of neglecting the emotional component of human illness. In some cases the emotions will play a participatory role; in others they are primary. To neglect this dimension of illness pathology is as great an omission as to ignore the role of microorganisms in human illness.

What emotions could be so terrible as to induce the brain to subject someone to severe physical pain and frightening neurological symptoms? The answer to this question is basic not only to the understanding of these pain syndromes but to the whole range of psychosomatic disorders.

Conflicts rage constantly in the unconscious, born of the various elements that represent the mosaic of the human psyche. These conflicts result in the development of emotions that cannot be tolerated and, therefore, must be repressed. Because these undesirable feelings appear to strive for recognition, the mind must do something to prevent them from coming to consciousness. Hence, the mindbody symptom. This book explores the nature and content of these undesirable feelings and explains why the mind chooses to mask emotional turmoil with physical pain.

The Mindbody Prescription

PART ONE

The Psychology and Physiology of Mindbody Disorders

1

The Psychology of
Mindbody Disorders:
A Tale of Two Minds

Since TMS and its equivalents are initiated by psychological
phenomena, an explanation of the psychology of mindbody
disorders is the logical place to begin. These disorders are
neither illnesses nor diseases, but rather symptomatic states
induced by the brain to serve a psychological purpose. I think
you will be able to relate to some of the following scenarios.

You are a single woman in your twenties or thirties. You
may or may not have an advanced degree, but you're trying
to make your way in your chosen field. Your family history
may be good, indifferent or distinctly bad, but you can think
of childhood recollections that are uncomfortable or painful.
Your love life, straight or gay, is not the best and you are concerned about whether or not to marry or establish a long-
term relationship. You wonder whether or not you want a
family. You may be having money problems. In a variety of
ways, a parent or parents (sometimes a sibling) may be a concern to you.

You are under pressure from these many life realities. To
make matters worse, you are driven by a strong need to make
it all work out, perfectly if possible, and/or a strong compulsion to be a "good" person, someone everybody likes, someone they can count on to help when trouble comes.

Perhaps you are the same age as this woman but you're married. Your marriage may vary from quite good to terrible, but in any case being married has added a large number of pressures you didn't have before. You're finding it harder to put in the time necessary to advance in your field. Even staying in shape has become a challenge. If the marriage is rocky, the stress is greater. Do you try to keep it together? Have you chosen the wrong mate? Will you ever find the ideal mate? Time is passing and it may be getting too late to have children.

Now complicate it further. You have one or more children. If you're a working woman the pressures are tremendous. Even if you're a stay-at-home mother, children change your life drastically, especially if you're a caring, conscientious mother. Should you stop working? What's best for the children? What's best for you? Paradoxically, children usually stress a marriage. Now there's much less time for the romance, fun and games, the carefree life of the young married couple. For parents of an infant a good night's sleep may be rare. Every year, parenthood creates new responsibilities, more restrictions on freedom. This applies to both parents, of course, unless the father is a chauvinist of the old school whose credo is, "The mother takes care of the children, I bring home the money."

You may be from a cultural tradition where large families are the rule, and five, six, seven or eight children are common. You love the idea, you have never felt burdened, but for some strange reason you have begun to have back pain. (You happen to be a meticulous person and a great worrier.)

Why do these scenarios refer only to life's negative aspects? The psychological reality is that while we all tend to make the best of things consciously, life's pressures produce internal reactions in the unconscious, of which we are totally unaware. We remain unaware of them even when they become disturbing enough to elicit physical symptoms. The realm of emotions contains two minds: the familiar conscious mind and the unconscious mind, a never-never land that actually has a more profound influence on our lives, on what we do or don't do, than its conscious counterpart. Although most people think decision making is the domain of the conscious mind, actually it is a process that draws upon all that has been learned and felt in the past, including information that resides in the unconscious.

Moving the clock ahead a few decades: You are now in your late forties, fifties or sixties. Children have grown up and departed; you may experience a loss of purpose and importance. If your marriage has not been good, it may further deteriorate, leaving you feeling trapped, wanting to leave but not daring to for a variety of reasons, often economic. You begin to wonder whether you have lived a full life. And, strange as it may seem, strong negative feelings about your mother or father have not gone away; instead, they continue to be repressed and may give rise to symptoms.

You may never have had a child and may, at a deep emotional level, feel very deprived, to such an extent that you develop symptoms.

Elderly parents may require much attention, inevitably evoking prodigious amounts of internal anger, of which you will be completely unaware. Despite your genuine love for your mother or father, the unconscious anger will come unbidden. When it reaches a critical level, symptoms will appear.

Retirement is generally "dangerous to your health," whether you're a man or a woman. The loss of status, the change of pattern and lifestyle almost invariably produce disturbing internal reactions that may cause emotional or physical symptoms.

Some of the strongest feelings arise in the nonworking wife of a retiree. Now you have to interact with your husband all his waking hours; you may find yourself cooking three meals a day. One woman remarked that it's like having a teenager around the house again.

If your husband gets sick, multiply the internal anger by ten. It doesn't matter how much you love him; the unconscious is not logical and is surely not thoughtful. If the marriage was a little rocky before his illness, it may be worse. after, adding to your internal rage.

You're a young unmarried man, out of school and finding it very hard to secure a suitable job. Or you've got a good job but it's a real pressure cooker. You're working long hours, doing a good job, but there's no promotion in sight. Maybe you're not making enough to live on your own so you have to stay with your parents, and that's a real pain because of problematic relations with your father (or mother, or sister, or brother).

Women may be a problem, or at least finding someone with whom you are comfortable. At times you date women who are really not suited to you, yet your strong need to be liked and accepted means you settle for less than the best. Because you feel inadequate, you accept low-level jobs below your capacity. Deep down inside you feel that you're not worth very much. That is enraging.

Or you're gay. Your partner is HIV positive. Or you haven't got a lover and you wish you could find one. You're not out of the closet; neither your boss nor your parents know; maybe you're not sure yourself.

Or you're in your mid-thirties, married with two small children, you own a small business or you work for a corporation. You're very successful but you've always been a worrier, even as a kid. You're extremely sensitive, easily hurt, expecting to be hurt or injured; you always put yourself down; you feel you must be liked by everybody and will put yourself out for anyone who asks for help, then find yourself wondering whether you did enough, were "good" enough. You always feel as though you have to prove yourself. You know you're anxious; you've had panic attacks. Strangely, very few people know this about you because you look and act very strong. Physically you're quite imposing.

You may have always been very active physically: tennis, running, basketball, volleyball, skiing. You've been married several years, have no children, work in advertising or a law firm. Your boss is a martinet and has you constantly uptight. Your wife wants to start a family but you're not sure it's the right time. A year ago you developed a little back pain; an MRI revealed a herniated disc. Now you're afraid to engage in any of the sports you loved and you're getting very depressed.

Maybe you're approaching fifty. You have been very successful, you're financially secure, but you find yourself constantly engaging in new projects, new challenges. You seem unable to relax and enjoy your achievements. You're beginning to get physical symptoms.

You've been a golfer all your life and you love the game. Your wife decided it would be nice if you could play a sport together. Because golf is of no interest to her, she suggested tennis. You've been trying to learn the game to please her but you're not good at it and you really don't like it. After many years your back has started to hurt again.

Or you've been working at the same plant for twenty years. You're good at your job but you've got a new superintendent who bugs you and won't let you make decisions. In addition, he keeps asking you to do things that should be assigned to the younger, less experienced men. These days you don't feel so well physically.

Coincidentally, that young man in your department who has been on the job for about a year seems to be having a lot of trouble with his neck and arms; he's been out sick quite a bit for the past few months. Talking to him, you've formed the impression that he hates the job but is staying on because the money's good. He's married and has three children.

You're seventy. A year ago, against your vote, your family sold the business to which you devoted your life. They were the financial brains but you were the technical genius who created the business. You've had terrible hip pain for the last six months that the doctors can't seem to figure out. It's getting so you can't walk more than a couple of blocks before it gets so bad you have to stop.

These brief sketches will not have described every reader's life. They are meant to highlight one of the primary messages of this book: We are all under one kind of pressure or another. We all have internal reactions to those pressures, and all of us will have physical symptoms in response to those inner feelings. No matter how we react to life's pressures consciously, another world of reactions exists in the unconscious. Because we are not aware of those unconscious feelings and cannot, therefore, control them, and because they are so threatening and frightening, the brain will automatically induce physical symptoms to prevent the dangerous feelings from becoming overt, and thus becoming conscious. That is how mindbody symptoms come about—and they are universal in Western society. They are not a sign of mental or emotional illness. To look upon them as abnormal or aberrant leads to gross medical mismanagement.

The Architecture of the Emotional Mind (Psyche)

Sigmund Freud developed the concepts of the unconscious and the repression of emotions in the unconscious. I believe psychogenic physical disorders (that is, disorders induced by emotions) develop because of undesirable or frightening repressed feelings. My theories, therefore, are rooted in fundamental psychoanalytic concepts. I have no psychoanalytic training and had no preconceived idea of the psychological nature of these disorders when I began to study the problem. It soon became apparent, however, that the symptom complexes under study were the result of a process that began in what psychologists call the unconscious, that part of the emotional domain of which we are totally unaware, and that physical symptoms were a reaction to unconscious feelings. Therefore, as with so much in the worlds of psychology and psychiatry, without Freud we might still be searching for an explanation. If he had not introduced the idea of repression in the unconscious we would have to attribute the symptoms to "nerves" and have no idea how to proceed therapeutically.

Freud conceived of three components of the emotional mind that his translators called the superego, the ego and the id. Transactional psychoanalysts refer to these components as parent, adult and child. For the purpose of teaching my theories I prefer the latter.

The parent is that part of the mind that tells us what is right and wrong, how we must behave and act morally and ethically. This parent resides in both the conscious and unconscious minds and plays a crucial role in psychogenic physical disorders. It is synonymous with conscience; the parent makes us perfectionists and what I term "goodists." A goodist has a compulsion to please, to be a good person, to be nice. A goodist avoids confrontation, is the peacemaker, always on the alert to help someone, even if it means self-sacrifice. The goodist has a great need to be liked, coupled with the fear of being disliked.

The perfectionist is hardworking, conscientious, responsible, achievement- and success-oriented, a worrier. The ultra-perfectionist is not content to be preeminent in his or her field and compulsively searches for new challenges.

The adult also functions in both the conscious and unconscious. It is the mediator, the executive, the captain of the ship. Its role is to keep you functioning optimally and protect you from external as well as internal dangers. The unconscious adult may react automatically to certain situations; hence, its decisions are not always logical or rational, according to conscious judgment. This tendency for irrationality in unconscious mental function is crucial to understanding mindbody disorders. The realm of the emotions is composed of two minds; too often we experience the dominance of the unconscious over the conscious. TMS and its equivalents are examples of that dominance.

Last, there is the child, the part of the mind we do not acknowledge but that plays a critical role in our daily lives. It is all unconscious, of course, or we would be constantly embarrassed. Like a real child, it is pleasure-oriented, entirely self-involved, dependent, irresponsible, charming, often illogical and irrational, but unlike a real child, perpetually angry. It is also powerful, although it sees itself as weak and inferior—"after all, I'm only a child." It is in constant conflict with the parent—a struggle of major importance to the mindbody process.

The concepts advanced by Heinz Kohut, a prominent twentieth-century psychoanalyst, are essential to understanding the sequence of events that lead to physical symptoms. Rather than speak of the child, Kohut postulated the existence of a self in each of us that develops poorly or well in the early months of life. He believed that self-involvement, technically known as *narcissism*, is normal and healthy if it develops properly, since narcissism characterizes a more or less cohesive self. He theorized a developmental line for narcissism, from the primitive to the fully mature. According to Kohut, narcissism is never given up, is potentially healthy and in a good environment develops into mature forms of self-esteem.

However, it was Kohut's reference to what he called narcissistic rage that particularly interested me. He postulated that people with personality disorders emerged from childhood with an accumulated, permanent rage that he called narcissistic rage. He suggested that emotional trauma experienced during the developmental years of infancy and childhood was responsible for this rage. I wondered whether there might be some of this rage in all of us, but more particularly, whether it was pressure on this inherently narcissistic self residing in each of us that produced the anger-rage that seems to be responsible for mindbody disorders. This idea is developed more fully in the section that follows.

With this background we can now examine precisely what goes on in the unconscious that leads to physical symptoms.

Pressure and Rage in the Unconscious

I believe that rage in the unconscious has three potential sources:

1. That which may have been generated in infancy and childhood and never dissipated
2. That which results from self-imposed pressure, as in driven, perfectionist or goodist people
3. That which is a reaction to the real pressures of everyday life

I find the analogy of a bank account helpful in describing this to patients. Deposits of anger are made not only during childhood but throughout a person's life. Because there are no withdrawals from this account, the anger accumulates. Thus anger becomes rage; when it reaches a critical level and threatens to erupt into consciousness, the brain creates pain or some other physical symptom as a distraction, to prevent a violent emotional explosion.

The following case history is a graphic and dramatic demonstration of this process. Only a small proportion of patients with TMS have histories as severe and upsetting as this one. However, I use this patient's experience because it makes the relationship between pain and repressed feelings crystal clear.

A Letter from Helen

I had successfully treated Helen for low back pain a number of months prior to the event described in her letter. When Helen was forty-seven, she remembered having been sexually abused by her father as a child and teenager. She decided to join a support group for adult women survivors of incest. The day of the first meeting her back began to hurt, but having been through my program she reassured herself that she knew the psychological reason for the pain and was not concerned. Her own words describe best what happened next:

"I went to the meeting, met the six other women, trying to keep kind of under control and not be totally emotional and miserable with people I had barely met. I wanted to see if this kind of group was really right for me. I found myself, in spite of trying to keep some distance, very much overwhelmed—by the amount of pain and havoc wrought in these women's lives, as well as my own, by the abuse."

Over the next forty-eight hours the pain gradually increased in severity to the point where she could not get out of bed: She was paralyzed with pain. She told her supportive husband that she couldn't understand why she should have this pain when she understood its psychogenic purpose. Distraught, she wondered why the therapeutic concept wasn't working.

He replied, "You're talking about forty years of repressed anger." This is what she wrote about what happened next:

"And then, in an instant, I started to cry. Not little tears, not sad, quiet oh-my-back-hurts-so-much tears, but the deepest, hardest tears I've ever cried. Out of control tears, anger, rage, desperate tears. And I heard myself saying things like, Please take care of me, I don't ever want to have to come out from under the covers, I'm so afraid, please take care of me, don't hurt me, I want to cut my wrists, please let me die, I have to run away, I feel sick—and on and on, I couldn't stop and R——, bless him, just held me. And as I cried, and as I voiced these feelings, it was, literally, as if there was a channel, a pipeline, from my back and out through my eyes. I FELT the pain almost pour out as I cried. It was weird and strange and transfixing. I knew—really knew—that what I was feeling at that moment was what I felt as a child, when no one would or could take care of me, the scaredness, the grief, the loneliness, the shame, the horror. As I cried, I was that child again and I recognized the feelings I have felt all my life which I thought were crazy or at the very best, bizarre. Maybe I removed myself from my body and never even allowed myself to feel when I was young. But the feelings were there and they poured over me and out of me."

I am grateful to Helen (whose name has been changed) for allowing me to print parts of her letter; they illustrate perfectly the process behind TMS and equivalent physical reactions. Her story demonstrates these critical points:

1. Feelings generated in infancy and childhood permanently reside in the unconscious and may be responsible for psychological and physical symptoms throughout life.

2. Strong, painful, embarrassing and threatening feelings, like rage, grief and shame, are repressed in the unconscious.

3. Repressed emotions constantly strive to come to consciousness—that is, escape from the unconscious and become overt and consciously manifest.

4. The purpose of symptoms, physical or emotional, is to prevent repressed feelings from becoming conscious by diverting attention from the realm of the emotions to that of the physical. It is strategy of avoidance.

Helen's story illustrates all four points. In less than two days her pain increased in severity despite her knowledge of its source. From her knowledge of TMS she was aware that understanding what was being repressed would usually abort the pain. In this case, it did not because the powerful, painful, threatening feelings continued to come closer and closer to breaking through to consciousness. As they did, the pain increased in a desperate attempt to prevent the breakthrough. The feelings would not be denied expression, *and when they exploded into consciousness the pain disappeared*. It no longer had a purpose; it had failed in its mission.

In virtually every case the brain's strategy does not fail; it succeeds in keeping the feelings repressed, and the pain persists. However, the psychotherapists who work with me relate that reactions like Helen's, though not as dramatic, occasionally occur in the course of effective therapy. As with Helen, the pain disappears immediately in consequence of the emotional experience.

It would save a lot of time and trouble if all my patients could have such a breakthrough. Because they do not and I do not know how to induce it, we must follow a more laborious procedure to banish the pain. The average patient with

TMS does not harbor the same degree of rage and, therefore, does not explode as Helen did.

Unconscious Rage and Unbearable Feelings: The Hidden Culprits

In reality, we have three minds: the conscious, the unconscious and the subconscious. This book is concerned primarily with the first two. The third, the subconscious, is the realm of perception, cognition, language production and comprehension, reason, judgment, physical and instrumental skill and the wellspring of creativity. It is a fascinating area but is relevant here only to the extent that learning takes place in the subconscious, and learning is the foundation of the therapeutic process.

Understanding the mindbody process requires some knowledge of the unconscious mind. I have laid some of the groundwork in the description of the parent, adult and child that reside in the unconscious. The following table may be helpful:

The Conscious Mind	The Unconscious Mind
External	Internal
Logical	Irrational
Thoughtful	Emotional
Controlled	Wild
Mature	Childish
Concerned for others	Self-involved, narcissistic
Strives to be perfect	Feels imposed upon—rage
Strives to be good	Feels imposed upon—rage
Guilty	Unconcerned
Courageous	Fearful
Independent	Dependent
Self-confident	Low self-esteem

Civilized	Savage
Moral	Amoral

The unconscious is not all negative, as the table might suggest. We are merely drawing attention to those qualities of the unconscious that lead to physical symptoms. The conscious mind copes very well with personality-imposed pressures and the pressures of daily life. It is the internal reactions to these pressures that lead to accumulated rage, and the threat that the rage will erupt into consciousness that necessitates a physical ailment as a distraction. Rage in the unconscious is perceived as dangerous and threatening by the unconscious, hence the dramatic overreaction in the form of pain and other physical symptoms.

To avoid any confusion it is essential to clarify the important difference between anger or rage we feel consciously and the repressed emotion referred to here.

Contemporary medical research on the relationship of emotions to pain, particularly chronic pain, focuses exclusively on what can be called *perceived emotions*. This includes such feelings as anger, anxiety, fear and depression. The person who suffers these feelings is aware of them; they are not repressed in the unconscious.

In my experience these may aggravate but they do not cause pain. TMS teaches us that only feelings that the mind perceives as dangerous, and therefore represses, induce physical reactions.

The Suppression of Conscious Anger

A very important book, *The Rage Within*, was published in 1984 by the noted psychoanalyst and author Willard Gaylin. It is a scholarly and insightful account of the causes and universal effects of anger and rage in the modern era. Dr. Gaylin makes it clear that suppressing anger is a fact of everyday life and, therefore, a psychosocial problem of great magnitude.

Inhibited or consciously suppressed anger contributes to the reservoir of rage in the unconscious. My work has dealt with pain disorders that are the *direct result* of anger-rage repressed (unconscious) and suppressed (conscious). While anger that is known to a person plays a role in the genesis of TMS when it is suppressed, it is not nearly as important as anger that is generated in the unconscious as a result of:

1. Internal conflict
2. Stresses and strains of daily life
3. The residue of anger from infancy and childhood

Moreover, people treated for TMS consistently get better; the same cannot be said for those treated for chronic pain in the medical community at large.

Rage—Not Anger

The intensity of the anger, to the point of rage, determines the necessity for physical symptoms as a diversion. The threat of rage to explode into consciousness must be of sufficient magnitude to warrant the production of TMS or one of its equivalents.

How Do You Know Rage Is the Culprit?

Throughout my experience with mindbody disorders, patients have been my source of information. I have learned by observing. Further, our psychologists repeatedly find evidence of repressed sadness and rage, and unconscious fear of these feelings. Helen is a prime example.

Examples abound, such as the man whose family sold, over his objection, a business that was his pride and joy; the man who felt compelled to participate in activity he dislikes to please his wife; the dozens of men and women looking after elderly parents, not objecting consciously, but seething inwardly; the young men and women who, like Helen, were sexually abused as children; the woman with six children who loves being a mother but is unaware of her inner anger at all that motherhood entails; the mother who invariably has a pain attack after holidays because of the enormous amount of work she had to do for the family, taken for granted by everyone; the fifty-five-year-old man who has been angry at his mother or father since childhood.

To varying degrees, I believe we all harbor repressed rage, that to do so is normal for our time and culture. We are all under pressure of one kind or another. Though it is well to be aware of this unconscious rage, it is equally important to focus on the sources of the rage. Before we do, a word about avoidance.

Avoidance: Symptom as a Distraction

As noted in the introduction, Stanley Coen, a Columbia psychoanalyst and author, suggested that the purpose of the pain was to distract attention from frightening, threatening emotions and to prevent their expression. It was crucial to understanding how emotions are related to physical symptoms and, as will be seen in the treatment chapter, why knowledge can banish symptoms.

Symptoms are not physical substitutes for bad feelings, like anxiety. Nor are they self-punishment for bad thoughts or guilt. They are players in a strategy designed to keep our attention focused on the body so as to prevent dangerous feelings from escaping into consciousness or to avoid confrontation with feelings that are unbearable.

Helen's experience represents a combination of both. She was enraged and shamed by the degradation of sexual abuse.

She harbored feelings of horror, loneliness, grief and fear, none of which was allowed into consciousness. However, stimulated by the support group, these feelings began to push ineluctably toward consciousness; as they did, the distracting pain increased in severity in a desperate attempt to prevent the eruption.

Because the unconscious is often illogical and irrational, it may react automatically in the face of disturbing feelings. Most people, if given the choice between coming to terms with difficult feelings or experiencing intense physical pain, would choose to deal with the feelings. That's logical. But the way the human emotional system is now organized dictates how it will react; at the unconscious level it is often illogical. If the brain continues to evolve, the unconscious may some-day be more rational. At the moment it is strongly influenced by childish, illogical reactions.

To understand the phenomenon of avoidance in TMS one must constantly bear in mind how radically the uncon-scious mind differs from its conscious counterpart. The un-conscious is terrified by the rage and reacts to avoid it by keeping it repressed and employing physical symptoms to aid in that repression. One of Freud's biographers, Peter Gay, likened the unconscious to a maximum-security prison where all the desperate criminals, the undesirables and unac-ceptables, are incarcerated under heavy lock and key. In other words, they are repressed.

If these feelings are already repressed, you may ask, what is the need for a distraction? The prison analogy is particu-larly apt; the repressed feelings, like desperadoes, will try to escape. Despite the force of repression, powerful emotions like rage *will strive to rise to consciousness*. I call it the "drive to consciousness." Yale philosopher-psychoanalyst Jonathan Lear refers to it as a "yearning for expression" and a desire for a "conscious unification of thought and feeling."

In *Beyond the Pleasure Principle,* Freud wrote, "The unconscious itself has no other endeavor than to break through the pressure weighing down on it and force its way either to consciousness or to a discharge through some real action."

Therapeutic experience lends further support to the concept. When patients become aware of the presence of rage or unbearable feelings, these feelings can cease their struggle to become conscious. Removing that threat eliminates the need for physical distraction, and the pain stops.

Rage seems to be the principal player in the syndrome of TMS. However, all strongly objectionable or unbearable feelings will be repressed and, since they are all trying to come to consciousness, may stimulate physical symptoms. This includes internal conflicts of all kinds, many of which require the expertise of a psychotherapist to unravel. Strong dependency needs, conflicts over sexuality, identity problems, feelings of helplessness, humiliation and shame do not usually come to my attention in my interaction with a patient. If these conflicts are at the root of continuing symptoms, psychotherapy is usually necessary to reverse the process.

The principle that physical symptoms serve as a distraction from unconscious phenomena has been important in understanding the nature of the mindbody process and, therefore, in the development of a therapeutic program. That basic idea has been validated by many years of successful treatment.

The Sources of Rage

This may be the most important subject in the entire mindbody process. Although awareness of the existence of rage in the unconscious is essential, to focus on it alone is not enough. We must seek to know the reasons for the rage to fully understand the process.

Trauma in Infancy and Childhood

Experiences in infancy and childhood make the earliest contribution to the pool of anger. Helen's story gives a painfully graphic example of what is unquestionably the most serious type of childhood emotional trauma: sexual abuse. Physical and emotional abuse can be almost as crippling to the psychological development of the child.

Emotional abuse may occur in the guise of "training." Strict rules of behavior, such as "Children should be seen and not heard" or "Nice little boys and girls don't have temper tantrums," and rigid ideas of right and wrong (religious training may impose this) are familiar examples. In addition, children of parents with significant psychological problems like alcoholism, drug addiction, depression, anxiety or psychosis often suffer lasting trauma.

If a mother is psychologically inadequate the delicate processes of mother-child bonding and establishing emotional independence, both of which occur in the first months of life, may be disturbed. If a mother was very dependent on her own mother, she may have a need to tie the child to herself because it makes her feel more secure. She may use the love of the child to substitute for the absence of love from her husband or her parents. Similarly, the father plays an important role in childhood development. He must be a model for the boy and the precursor of a lover for the girl. If he decides that bringing up children is the woman's job, his children are in trouble. Either parent can have exalted expectations for their children—such as academic, athletic or artistic—creating great pressures that may not be bearable.

Unconscious resentments may occur in perfectly normal settings. One need not postulate "bad," "cruel" or "inadequate" parents.

Deeply repressed feelings of inadequacy foster the development of personality traits that are almost universal in people with TMS. They tend to be perfectionistic, compulsive, highly conscientious and ambitious; they are driven, self-critical and generally successful. Parallel with these traits, and sometimes more prominent, is the compulsion to please, to be a good person, to be helpful and nonconfrontational. In short, people with TMS have a strong need to seek approval, whether it is love, admiration or respect.

What's wrong with being perfect and good? Nothing at all from the standpoint of society and career, but the negative unconscious consequences can be extremely important.

Personality Traits

LOW SELF-ESTEEM

Low self-esteem is so pervasive in our society that one is inclined to invoke both genetic and developmental factors.

Deeply repressed feelings of inadequacy and self-doubt appear to be our common lot. Earlier societies may have done a better job of rearing their offspring by being more nurturing, less controlling, having a simpler set of rules by which to live and providing good role models and rites of passage.

That we all harbor inner feelings of inadequacy cannot be proven, but modern psychoanalytic theorists, like Kohut, have suggested that faulty development of the inner self early in life leaves us with unconscious childish feelings in an adult world.

PERFECTIONISM

The drive to be perfect must surely derive from a deep need to demonstrate to ourselves and to the world that we are truly worth something. Virtually every patient I have seen in the course of my experience with pain syndromes has been to a greater or lesser degree perfectionistic. Patients who deny it then go on to describe how they are very fussy about neatness, cleanliness and other aspects of their lives. If they do not admit to being perfectionistic, they acknowledge that they are highly responsible, conscientious, concerned and prone to worry. They are usually ambitious, hard-driving and self-critical; they set high standards of performance and behavior for themselves. An inner sense of inadequacy fuels perfectionism. A person's station in life or achievements are often deceiving. Feelings of inadequacy are deeply unconscious and, paradoxically, often drive us to be very successful.

Why does the drive to be perfect lead to rage? The pressure superimposed by the mind-parent on the residual child is enraging. Ben Sorotzkin, a practicing psychologist, suggests that perfectionists unconsciously set up standards for themselves they cannot possibly meet; their inevitable failure to live up to them results in unconscious shame and rage.

GOODISM

Perfectionism is the predominant personality characteristic in many of my patients. In others, however, a closely related compulsion—the need to be good—is primary. These people are driven to be helpful, often to the extent of sacrificing their own needs. They have a desire to ingratiate, to want everyone to like them. Cultural or religious influences can enhance this tendency. Society mandates that you be a good son or daughter, a good spouse, a good parent, a congenial fellow-worker. This powerful drive, like perfectionism, seems to stem from deep feelings of inadequacy.

What's wrong with striving to be perfect and good? Doesn't that benefit everybody? From a social and interpersonal perspective, it's wonderful, but it also engenders great internal anger. Though we may consciously want to be and do good, the narcissistic self does not have such an imperative. Indeed, it reacts with anger at the imposition. Add to this the unconscious anger at not being fully appreciated for our efforts and, worst of all, the anger at ourselves for not living up to our own expectations.

Remember, the unconscious is often irrational. A young mother with a newborn, whom she loves dearly, is very worried about doing things right, and she's up half the night. Completely preoccupied with being a mother, she is unaware that she is unconsciously angry at the baby. Many of my patients have found it difficult to accept the idea that parents may be unconsciously angry at their children.

HOSTILITY AND AGGRESSION

Much has been written about the potential danger of hostility and aggression to our health. Hostility is said to be the most important of the so-called Type A behavior traits related to coronary arteriosclerosis. Once again, focus is on perceived emotions. TMS theory would identify hostility and aggression as overt manifestations of something far more dangerous—repressed rage and suppressed anger. Physical symptoms, anxiety, depression or hostility are, in effect, equivalents of each other. They all reflect powerful processes going on in the unconscious.

GUILT

Recently a patient was describing her compulsion to please and be a good person. "Not only that," she added, "but I feel so guilty about not being good or kind enough or doing enough for the people in my life."

Guilt is another reaction spawned by the psychic parent, another self-imposed pressure that contributes to the critical mass of rage. One can feel guilty about many things, including past transgressions and inadequacies. Because the self cannot tolerate discomfort of any kind, and guilt is yet another attack on our sense of worth, all contribute to the rage. Self-criticism is apparently as enraging as criticism from others.

DEPENDENCY

One of the residuals of childhood is the desire to be taken care of. Because we do not view this desire as appropriate adult behavior, it is deeply repressed; we are unconsciously dependent. This may lead to unconscious anger because the dependency needs are never satisfied and, paradoxically, we may be unconsciously angry at the person or persons upon whom we are dependent.

Unconscious dependency may lead to other angering complications, such as the poor choice of a mate (someone who will "mother" us) or choosing a profession or work that will be secure or without responsibility, though neither challenging nor fulfilling. Other reactions to the deep-seated feelings of dependency are fierce independence and even aggression.

Understanding the impact of low self-esteem, perfectionism, goodism, guilt and dependency supports the idea that rage is the emotion primarily implicated in the development of mindbody symptoms in disorders like TMS. Feelings of inadequacy and dependency lead to perfectionistic, people-pleasing, guilty-producing propensities. The self, like a child, reacts to the pressure. A circular process is at work here: The self stimulates personality traits that, in turn, anger the self.

The World Around Us

Pressure is enraging to the self, whether it is pressure from within at the dictates of the parent or from the realities of our daily lives. Being conscientious and concerned makes matters worse, aggravating the pressure of being a competent worker, a good spouse and parent, a loving child to an elderly, dependent parent.

Even happy events like landing a good job, getting married or having a baby can result in inner turmoil, pressure and anger. Many young mothers who began having back pain during their pregnancies were in conflict about their adequacy as mothers or ambivalent about having interrupted their careers to have a baby.

At the other end of the emotional spectrum, the inner self, feeling abandoned, may react with anger at a loved one who dies or a child who leaves home.

Many years ago New York psychiatrists Thomas Holmes and Richard Rahe studied the causative role of stressful life events "in the natural history of many diseases." They reported on a list of these events, some of which were negative but many identified as socially desirable and "consonant with the American values of achievement, success, materialism, practicality, efficiency, future orientation, conformism and self-reliance." The list is reproduced here. We postulate that these events produce "disease" through the mechanism of internal rage. The events are listed in order of decreasing stress:

1. Death of a spouse
2. Divorce
3. Marital separation
4. Jail term
5. Death of close family member
6. Personal injury or illness
7. Marriage
8. Fired at work
9. Marital reconciliation
10. Retirement

11. Change in health of family member
12. Pregnancy
13. Sex difficulties
14. Gain of a new family member
15. Business readjustment
16. Change in financial state
17. Death of a close friend
18. Change to different line of work
19. Change in number of arguments with spouse
20. Mortgage over $10,000 [in the 1960s]
21. Foreclosure of mortgage or loan
22. Change of responsibilities at work
23. Son or daughter leaving home
24. Trouble with in-laws
25. Outstanding personal achievement
26. Wife begins or stops work
27. Begin or end school
28. Change in living conditions
29. Revision of personal habits
30. Trouble with boss
31. Change in work hours or conditions
32. Change in residence
33. Change in schools
34. Change in recreation
35. Change in church activities
36. Change in social activities
37. Mortgage or loan less than $10,000
38. Change in sleeping habits
39. Change in number of family get-togethers
40. Change in eating habits
41. Vacation
42. Christmas
43. Minor violations of the law

Both positive and negative stress generate unconscious anger, whether or not one is consciously angry. Accumulated anger is rage, and frightening, unconscious rage leads to the development of physical symptoms.

Six Basic Needs

To fulfill our basic needs we put ourselves under pressure, which is enraging to the self. Or we become frustrated and angry because some of the needs are not adequately met. These basic needs are:

1. To be perfect (to excel, achieve, succeed; high expectations and standards; self-critical and very sensitive to criticism)
2. To be liked (approved of, loved, admired, respected; a compulsion to please, be a "nice guy," or be a mother or father to the world)
3. To be taken care of (a desire that never goes away unconsciously no matter how old or independent we are)
4. To be soothed (so we seek gratification through food, drink, smoking, sex, entertainment, play)
5. To be physically invincible (strong, unrestricted, sexy)
6. To be immortal (we are unconsciously enraged by the inevitability of death)

This last category is sometimes one of the most subtle. However, it is often responsible for the onset of pain in men and women in their fifties, sixties and seventies. Aging is enraging, something I had never thought about until I experienced it. Some of my patients have been aware of it but most did not realize the intensity of their inner feelings on the subject.

The Rage/Soothe Ratio

I believe a kind of rage/soothe ratio may play a role in determining when physical symptoms will occur. Patients frequently ask, "Why did the pain start now?" Invariably I reply, "Because your rage has reached a critical level; because it now threatens to erupt into consciousness."

Suppose, however, there is another element in the equation; that it is not simply the quantity of rage that brings on symptoms, but the presence or absence of counterbalancing soothing factors. Theoretically, these pleasant elements in a person's life would modify the threat posed by the rage and make symptoms unnecessary. One can carry this to the point of absurdity, but I believe something like it goes on and that the occurrence of symptoms reflects too much rage and not enough counteracting soothing elements in one's life.

The Concept of Equivalency

TMS is one of a group of interchangeable physical disorders. They all serve the same mindbody purpose and are, therefore, equivalents of each other. Indeed, any physical disorder that attracts a person's attention—for example, a fracture or severe respiratory infection—may replace the mindbody process temporarily. The pain syndrome frequently disappears with the advent of some new condition, only to recur when it is gone.

In a survey done in 1975 it was found that 88 percent of patients with TMS had histories of up to five common mindbody disorders, including a variety of stomach symptoms, such as heartburn, acid indigestion, gastritis and hiatus hernia; problems lower in the gastrointestinal tract, such as spastic colon, irritable bowel syndrome and chronic constipation; common allergic conditions, such as hay fever and asthma; a variety of skin disorders, such as eczema, acne, hives and psoriasis; tension or migraine headache; frequent urinary tract or respiratory infections; and dizziness or ringing in the ears (not associated with neurologic or ear disease). Not everyone agrees that these are mindbody disorders but I have found them to be so in my clinical practice. They usually occurred in tandem, suggesting that they all served the same psychological purpose. The fact that they were so common in TMS patients is what inclined me to conclude that TMS was a mindbody malady, too.

Anxiety and Depression as Equivalents

The idea that the physical conditions just listed are psychologically induced is controversial. Even more controversial is my conclusion that both anxiety and depression are equivalents of TMS, signifying that they, too, may serve to distract us from underlying, threatening emotions. The psyche is eclectic in its choice of distractors.

The following case histories illustrate the equivalency of anxiety and depression.

The first concerns a single woman in her late forties who was totally disabled from long-term chronic low back pain. She had been exhaustively studied and treated, to no avail. There was nothing structurally wrong with her lower spine; her X rays showed the usual changes associated with aging. As she was basically normal on physical examination, I diagnosed Tension Myositis Syndrome.

The severity of her symptoms put her in the hospital. There she was treated with physical therapy, my education program and psychotherapy. She experienced a gradual but progressive alleviation of pain. One morning she came into my office to tell me that the pain was gone but that she had become extremely anxious, to such an extent that she almost wished she could have her pain back. Having lost the pain as distraction, the brain substituted an anxiety state.

I believe depression can operate the same way.

One of my patients was a fifty-year-old man who had been treated successfully for various manifestations of TMS over a period of years. He also had a long history of depression, for which he was treated with medications and psychotherapy. Early in 1994 he was put on an antidepressant that was very effective and by the fall he was in excellent spirits. At this point he suddenly developed severe manifestations of TMS, including major muscle weakness in one of his ankles. I interpreted this as a case of symptom substitution. The medication had altered the brain chemistry and alleviated the depression, but it had done nothing to change the intrapsychic conflicts responsible for the depression. Therefore, another distraction had to be found and the mind resorted to one it had used many times before: back and leg pain.

Panic attacks (physical manifestations of acute anxiety) are also reactions to anger either repressed or suppressed. I recall a patient who said that he had been on the verge of lashing out at a woman about something, decided it would not be gentlemanly, suppressed the anger, and immediately experienced a panic attack. Other studies support this equivalency. One called chronic pain (TMS can become chronic) a pathological emotion, like anxiety and depression. Others have described chronic pain as psychologically equivalent to depression.

The Fear Factor

Fear is another important equivalent of pain that may be more effective than the pain itself to achieve the mind's goal of distracting attention from repressed rage. The *fear* of pain, physical activity, injury or spinal abnormality is enough to perpetuate TMS, even in the absence of pain. The mind is interested only in keeping our attention on the body; the fear of any of these phenomena will accomplish that as well as the reality of pain itself. This is why our therapeutic program requires not only the cessation of pain but the elimination of fear.

Obsessive-Compulsive Disorder as an Equivalent

A very intelligent, perceptive patient is largely responsible for this insight. He exhibited a classic case of TMS but did not mention that he had been suffering from obsessive-compulsive disorder (OCD) as well. OCD is characterized by the continuous performance of ritualistic acts, or thinking obsessive thoughts. It is both disturbing and functionally intrusive. A classic example is the hand-washing compulsion in which patients clean their hands hundreds of times a day because they are obsessed with a fear of germs. The drive to do or think these things is irresistible.

This patient decided that the psychology underlying TMS and OCD was the same and proceeded to apply the therapeutic principles of the former to the latter—with excellent results. In fact, his OCD disappeared before his back pain did.

OCD is an anxiety equivalent, which is a TMS equivalent. Hence, the decision to include OCD as a TMS equivalent is logical. Its capacity to absorb the patient's attention parallels that of the pain of TMS. Not infrequently, patients with TMS are obsessed with their pain symptoms, indicating the intensity of the unconscious need for a distraction.

Many of the theories I have suggested in this chapter are

controversial and will be disputed by people from many professional disciplines. They are the result of my clinical experience and since I am not trained in psychoanalysis, psychology or psychiatry may be questioned by these professionals. But it must be remembered that the field of mindbody medicine has not been studied with anywhere near the intensity in the latter half of this century as it was in the time of Freud and his followers. It has been almost totally neglected by physical medical specialties and psychiatry. Nonphysician psychologists are not trained to evaluate physical conditions and cannot, therefore, contribute to the study of the physical manifestations of these disorders. Physician psychoanalysts have been the only group to retain an interest in and continue to write on the subject, but their scope is limited, since they see only the most severe examples of mindbody disorders, like ulcerative colitis.

My psychological theories refer only to physical symptoms that are emotionally induced. I am not a psychotherapist, treating the emotional symptoms of psychological disorders. I am a physical doctor who has identified the psychological cause of a physical disorder. Therefore, what I propose must be evaluated in a different context from that of structurally oriented physical physicians, on the one hand, or psychologists-psychiatrists, on the other. We need a conceptual bridge. Let's see if we can construct it.

2

The Mechanics of
Mindbody Processes

The Mindbody Concept

This section is intended to be a bridge both organizationally and conceptually, linking emotional activity in the brain to physical symptoms in the body. The book began with a description of the emotional state believed to be responsible for many physical disorders and will continue, following this bridge, with a description of the disorders themselves.

Much has been written for the general public about the "mindbody" connection in the last twenty years. Authors such as Herbert Benson, Deepak Chopra, Norman Cousins, Dennis Jaffe, Lawrence LeShan, Steven Locke and Douglas Colligan, Joyce McDougall, Morton Reiser, Ernest Rossi, Bernie Siegel, Graeme Taylor and Andrew Weil, coming from a variety of backgrounds and disciplines, all share the conviction that the mind has the capacity to combat disease and improve health. There is no question that this is correct. What must be done, however, is to demonstrate scientifically how the mind can cause or cure physical maladies. This book presents a specific example of both those powers, describing how the brain creates the physical symptoms of the Tension Myositis Syndrome (TMS) and its equivalents, and how it can alleviate them.

The Status of Psychosomatic Medicine

Throughout the book I use the words *psychosomatic* and *mindbody* interchangeably. They are synonymous and refer to the interaction between the brain and the body whereby psychological or mental processes induce either pathological or beneficial physical changes. The word *psychosomatic* is widely misunderstood to describe an imaginary disorder experienced by people who are mentally abnormal, or an exaggeration of symptoms that are structurally based ("real"). To set the record straight, psychosomatic symptoms are real, they occur in normal people and they are universal in Western society.

Most of the literature on this subject refers to mind and body or the mind-body (hyphenated) connection. Candace Pert, who did basic research at the National Institutes of Health showing widespread and intimate connections between the brain and the body, first suggested that the words *mind* and *body* be joined. In view of my experience with TMS, I have adopted this usage.

In the introduction to his book *Psychosomatic Medicine*, published in 1950, Franz Alexander wrote: "Once again, the patient as a human being with worries, fears, hopes, and despairs, as an indivisible whole and not merely the bearer of organs—of a diseased liver or stomach—is becoming the legitimate object of medical interest. A growing psychological orientation manifests itself among physicians."

Ironically, the movement Alexander heralded almost died with him. The historical process upon which he commented, the dominance of technological, disease-oriented, antipsychological medicine, has continued and intensified so that very few people are carrying on the important work he began. Conventional medicine, including psychiatry, does not accept the theory presented in the previous chapter. It does not believe that emotions can initiate physical symptoms. The *Diagnostic and Statistical Manual of Mental Disorders*, the official list of psychiatric diagnoses of the American Psychiatric Association, does not use the word *psychosomatic*.

Alexander believed that emotional phenomena could initiate such physical disorders as stomach ulcers and TMS. He also studied the effect of emotional phenomena on the gastrointestinal tract, and on the respiratory, cardiovascular, endocrine, joint and muscle systems. He further believed that specific emotional states were responsible for each physical disorder.

By contrast, TMS theory states that the internal psychological process described in Chapter 1 is responsible for all psychogenic physical maladies, but with great variation in the details and severity of both the physiologic and psychological states.

Conventional medicine resists concepts like these even when presented with convincing evidence that they are valid. This reflects a deeply held philosophical bias that a "mindbody" interaction does not exist, on the one hand, and a conviction that laboratory science is the only valid science, on the other. Psychosomatic phenomena cannot be studied in the test tube or by using laboratory animals. Unconscious emotions are not revealed by the administration of tests or personality profiles.

The medical experience described in this book is an example of another kind of scientific method, in which diagnostic and therapeutic hypotheses are tested in large numbers of patients over many years. The fact that many people have "cured" themselves by a study of my books is in itself evidence of the accuracy of the TMS diagnosis. I have seen about ten thousand patients with TMS since 1973, most of whom have been rendered pain-free and fully physically active. This is science, too. Twenty-five years of experience with TMS in which there has been consistent, numerically impressive therapeutic success is more than a reasonable test of validity—it is proof of the accuracy of the diagnosis.

Stephen Jay Gould, who teaches biology, geology and the history of science at Harvard University, wrote an excellent defense of "soft science" in his June 1986 essay in *Natural History*:

> An unfortunate, but regrettably common, stereotype about science divides the profession into two domains of different status. We have, on the one hand, the "hard," or physical sciences that deal in numerical precision, prediction and experimentation. On the other hand, "soft" sciences that treat the complex objects of history in all their richness must trade these virtues for "mere" description without firm numbers in a confusing world where, at best, we can hope to explain what we cannot predict. The history of life embodies all the messiness of this second, and undervalued, style of science.

The study of human emotions and their consequences also falls into this "messy" category. It does not even share the relative neatness of historical science, with which Gould deals, for it does not yet possess the tools necessary to understand the basis for emotions.

Contemporary psychiatric research identifies chemical events in the brain associated with certain pathological states, like depression, and then assumes that if the symptom can be altered with drugs, the disorder is cured. TMS theory holds that depression and the chemical changes in the brain associated with depression are secondary to frightening feelings in the unconscious.

People who study the emotions and psychosomatic medicine must overcome the inferiority complex that stems from their inability to use the tools of "hard science." I refer to another Gould essay:

> This unnecessary humility follows an unfortunate tradition of self-hate among scientists who deal with the complex, unrepeatable and unpredictable events of history [substitute "the complex, poorly understood realm of human emotions"]. We are trained to think that the "hard science" models of quantification, experimentation and replication are inherently superior and exclusively canonical, so that any other set of techniques can only pale by comparison. But historical science proceeds by reconstructing a set of contingent events, explaining in retrospect what could not have been predicted beforehand. If the evidence be sufficient, the explanation can be as rigorous and confident as anything done in the realm of experimental science. In any case, this is the way the world works; no apologies needed.

There is a parallel between Gould's historical science and the science of mindbody disorders. Neither can make use of the laboratory but both can be studied rigorously. With TMS and its equivalents careful observation and replicable therapeutic experience are every bit as scientific as the concrete methods of quantification.

If one can banish a symptom through learning, the symptom must have originated in the brain. Since contemporary research maintains that all brain reactions, including those involving the emotions, can be identified chemically, perhaps we have succeeded in altering the brain's chemistry through learning.

The medical literature documents just such an observation, one that has been confirmed with a "hard science" method. In a study by Jeffrey Schwartz and his colleagues at the UCLA School of Medicine, patients with obsessive-compulsive disorder showed considerable improvement with cognitive-behavioral psychotherapy. Their symptomatic improvement was paralleled by a change toward normal on a measure of brain metabolic activity, the so-called PET (Positron Emission Tomography) scan.

Psychopharmacology, the branch of medicine that uses drugs in the treatment of psychological disorders, is guilty of very unscientific thinking when it asserts that it can cure an emotional disorder by altering the brain chemistry associated with that disorder. But that may be no more true than saying that the cause of pneumonia is fever. Identifying the chemistry of a clinical state is not establishing its cause. We may be looking at a result rather than a cause. If that is the case, treating depression with antidepressant drugs may be poor medicine for some patients: The symptom is being eliminated without identifying its cause.

Experience with TMS indicates that if an emotionally induced symptom is artificially removed with a drug or a placebo, one of two things will happen: The symptom will return when the drug is withdrawn or, more problematic, something will develop to take its place, either emotional or physical. The patient discussed in Chapter 1 got his depression under control with a medication, only to suffer a recurrence of his severe back pain, which he had previously eliminated.

Mindbody symptoms exist to serve a purpose. If you thwart that purpose by taking away the symptom without dealing with its cause, the brain will simply find a substitute symptom or disorder.

A Classification of Emotionally Induced Physical Disorders

Mindbody and *psychosomatic* are synonymous terms. In my previous books I did not use the term *psychosomatic* because people believe it means "imaginary" and that anyone with psychosomatic symptoms is weak or inadequate. I find this particularly ironic, since it appears that psychosomatic conditions are universal in Western society. We all have them; therefore, it is normal to have them. Remember:

1. Psychosomatic (mindbody) symptoms encompass a large number of common, harmless physical maladies like headache, stomachache, allergies and skin conditions.
2. We all experience one or more of them in the course of our lives.
3. They are not imaginary, foolish or hypochondriacal.
4. They are responsible for the epidemic of pain syndromes of various kinds that now afflict the Western world, including most back, neck, shoulder and limb pain, and many others to be described in Part II of this book.
5. These maladies have become public health problems because medicine does not recognize their emotional causation and is, therefore, incapable of dealing with them adequately.

The word that encompasses *all* emotionally induced physical disorders is *psychogenic*. A psychosomatic malady is a type of psychogenic manifestation. Following is a classification of psychogenic processes. I will explain each one:

1. Psychogenic regional (conversion, hysterical) disorders
2. Psychogenic intensification of symptoms
3. Psychogenic reduction or abolition of symptoms
4. Psychotic (delusional) symptoms
5. Psychosomatic (mindbody) disorders

Psychogenic Regional (Conversion, Hysterical) Disorders

Allan Walters, a Canadian neurologist, suggested using the term *psychogenic regional pain* in place of *hysterical pain*, the traditional term first used by Freud and his colleagues, since many patients were clearly not hysterics, though the cause of their pain was emotional. The term *conversion* was also used in Freud's time, implying that an emotional state had been converted into a physical one. In this category, emotional states bring about symptoms in the motor and sensory systems and organs of special senses without producing physiologic alteration in the body, as can be seen in Figure 1.

Figure 1
A Model for Psychogenic Regional (Conversion, Hysterical) Disorders

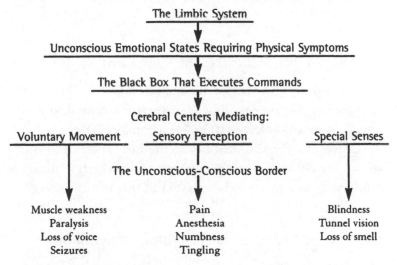

In this representation the limbic system encompasses all brain matter that generates emotions; the brain cells that comprise the limbic system are among the most important in that category. From these brain structures come the unconscious emotional states described in Chapter 1 that necessitate physical symptoms. The "black box" refers to that as yet unidentified part of the brain, and the process that goes on there, that stimulates activity in the cerebral (brain) centers that will produce one of a variety of abnormal reactions in the motor system, the sensory system or the special senses such as vision and hearing. These symptoms are perceived as a result of brain activity alone; there is no identifiable reaction in the body to account for them. They were common in Freud's time but are seen much less frequently now, probably because they are no longer in style.

Edward Shorter, a medical historian at the University of Toronto, made it quite clear in his book, *From Paralysis to Fatigue*, that mindbody symptom choice is based on what is in vogue at the time and what has been legitimized as "physical" by doctors.

Psychogenic Intensification of Symptoms

Fear or anxiety can make any symptom worse. This is the one psychogenic process that is generally accepted in medicine. It is usually referred to as "psychological overlay."

Unfortunately, this idea is also used to explain a disorder known as chronic pain, a concept with which I disagree strongly. This is discussed in Part II of this book.

Psychogenic Reduction or Abolition of Symptoms

This refers to a reduction or even abolition of a symptom such as pain. It is rarely encountered in civilian life, where pain and other symptoms are usually accompanied by varying degrees of emotional distress. By contrast, one of the earliest students of pain, Henry Beecher, observed during World

War II that severely wounded soldiers often required little or no morphine for pain control. The soldiers were so glad to be alive, though badly wounded, so relieved that they would not have to face the horror of the battlefield again and that they would now be taken care of, that they had little or no pain. Remarkable, and one more demonstration of the power of the mind. Injuries of similar magnitude in civilian life would be accompanied by great anxiety and the need for large doses of morphine.

Psychotic (Delusional) Symptoms

Like psychogenic regional symptoms, these are elaborated entirely in the brain as a result of serious mental illness. I have no experience with them but they are included here because they are psychogenic.

Psychosomatic (Mindbody) Disorders

These disorders, which will be described in Part II, include:

The Tension Myositis Syndrome (TMS)
Most low back and leg pain
Most neck, shoulder and arm pain
Possible cranial nerve pain or weakness (fifth and
      seventh cranial nerves)
Fibromyalgia
Tension myalgia
Myofascial pain syndrome
Temporomandibular joint syndrome
Most tendonitis syndromes
Carpal tunnel syndrome
Repetitive stress injury

Reflex sympathetic dystrophy
Post-polio syndrome
Most chronic pain
Most of those with so-called chronic fatigue syndrome
Most of those with the Epstein-Barr syndrome

The Equivalents of TMS

Gastrointestinal disorders
Disorders of the circulatory system
Skin disorders
Disorders of the immune system
Genitourinary disorders
Benign disorders of the cardiac mechanism
Miscellaneous disorders

Disorders in which Emotions May Play a Role

Autoimmune disorders
Cancer
Cardiovascular disorders

The Neurophysiology of Psychogenic Disorders

Here is the basic premise: Emotional states are capable of inducing physical symptoms, with or without physiologic alteration of specific tissues in the body.

Most contemporary medical practitioners, including
many psychiatrists, do not believe this occurs. In fact, medical
research is often at great pains to disprove psychogenic causation. A good example is the recent discovery that some people with peptic ulcers in the stomach harbor a bacterium,
Helicobacter pylori. Doctors have concluded that this bacterium, rather than stress, is the cause of ulcers.

The truth is that the presence of the bacterium does not

change the fact that emotional factors set the stage for the ulcer. I have had many patients who moved from musculoskeletal pain to pre-ulcer and ulcer symptoms and vice versa, with the emotional progenitors often clearly defined.

How Do Emotions Induce Physical Symptoms?

Because medical science has not yet unraveled the mystery of how the brain does what it does, we do not know the answer to this question. One might ask analogous questions that also defy explanation: How does the brain think, how does it produce and comprehend language, how does it create? In other words, at the most fundamental level we do not yet understand brain function. Medical science, therefore, cannot dismiss the idea that in addition to speech, cognition and creativity, the brain can also *cause* physical symptoms.

The Neurophysiology of Psychogenic Regional (Conversion, Hysterical) Disorders

In the study of psychogenic physical disorders, patients *are* the laboratory. Figure 1 (page 41) shows the process is initiated by an unconscious emotional state. The "black box" then stimulates areas of the brain that control voluntary movement and/or the perception of sensations coming in from the body or those that have to do with the special senses like vision, hearing, taste and smell. The crucial point is that the symptoms are not the result of damage or disease of specific body parts. They are perceived as weakness, pain, numbness or blindness only because the appropriate brain cells have been "fired off." That is known as a conversion reaction. One set of brain cells is stimulated to activity by other brain cells;

in this case, the stimulating cells are those having to do with powerful unconscious emotions.

Freud was the first to describe conversion symptoms, though he did not speculate on the brain process that might cause them. His recognition of the ability of emotional phenomena to induce physical symptoms stands as one of the most important scientific observations of the modern era.

Psychogenic regional symptoms produce no physiologic changes in the body. The entire process takes place in the cerebrum of the brain.

The Neurophysiology of Mindbody (Psychosomatic) Disorders

Figure 2 (page 47) shows that the preliminary process in the evolution of a mindbody disorder is the same as in a psychogenic regional malady. While some researchers have speculated that specific psychological states induce specific physical manifestations, that has not been my experience. My patients have shown that the underlying psychology is the same for conversion and mindbody disorders. It is as though the brain had decided that conversion symptoms were no longer convincing as disease, so it began to produce processes in which there were obvious physiologic alterations. This was done by involving the autonomic and immune systems in the production of symptoms. The part of the brain known as the hypothalamus is an essential way station in the process. The result is TMS and all the equivalents I have listed. Those symptoms resulting from immune system dysfunction reflect either too much or too little reaction to foreign invaders, like pollens or bacteria. Too much results in allergic reactions, too little in a susceptibility to illnesses such as frequent colds or urinary tract or yeast infections.

Figure 2
A Model for Mindbody (Psychosomatic) Disorders

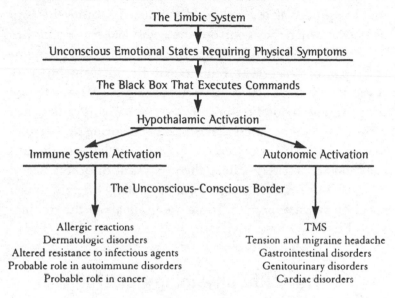

The Somatization Myth

In the *Diagnostic and Statistical Manual of Mental Disorders, Fourth Edition* (*DSM-IV*) the term *psychosomatic* does not appear in the section on physical symptoms of psychological origin. This is because most psychiatrists do not believe that emotions stimulate physiologic processes. They prefer the terms *somatization* and *somatoform disorder*.

Medical principles are thus established by majority fiat rather than by scientific evidence. Most psychiatrists reject the idea that unconscious phenomena lead to physical symptoms, hence the definition in *DSM-IV*; but that is precisely what my work has demonstrated. *DSM-IV* defines *somatization* as a "tendency to experience and communicate somatic distress and symptoms *unaccounted for by pathological findings*" [italics mine]. My patients would be irate at the suggestion that there was no real basis for their pain. They have real physical symptoms produced by a real pathophysiologic alteration of their muscles, nerves and tendons, and they know that the process is psychologically induced because the pain goes away when they confront the emotional reasons for it.

Rejection of the role of unconscious emotional phenomena is part of the current trend to bash Freud. Contemporary psychiatry (except for most psychoanalysts) prefers to use drugs and behavioral techniques to treat patients rather than get involved in the "messy" business of exploring the person's unconscious. This is extremely unfortunate because the unconscious is precisely where these physical disorders begin. The use of drugs and behavioral psychology merely puts a cover on an unsavory pot. It does nothing about the troublesome brew.

The Pathophysiology of TMS

Figure 3
The Pathophysiology of TMS

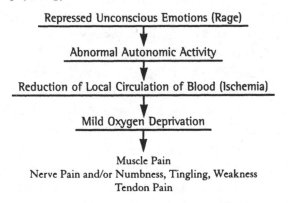

Repressed Unconscious Emotions (Rage)

↓

Abnormal Autonomic Activity

↓

Reduction of Local Circulation of Blood (Ischemia)

↓

Mild Oxygen Deprivation

↓

Muscle Pain
Nerve Pain and/or Numbness, Tingling, Weakness
Tendon Pain

Chapter 1 explained that the purpose of psychogenic symptoms is to draw attention away from emotional phenomena and focus it on the body. All of the mindbody disorders discussed in this book serve that purpose, but the various manifestations of TMS are far and away the most common.

How does the brain induce TMS?

Laboratory and clinical evidence suggest that it has chosen to work through the autonomic nervous system, the subsection of the central nervous system that controls the body's involuntary functions, including the circulation of blood. By mildly restricting the flow of blood to the target tissues, it reduces the available oxygen. The result is pain if muscle or tendon are the targets, and pain, numbness, tingling and perhaps weakness if a nerve is involved.

The theory of mild oxygen deprivation as the basis for symptoms was based on early observations that patients usually experienced temporary pain relief from physical therapy consisting of high-frequency sound waves, massage, and active exercise. Since all of these treatments tend to increase the local blood supply, reduced levels of oxygen seemed to be the culprit.

There has been some laboratory confirmation of this hypothesis. More than twenty years ago research workers observed microscopic evidence of mild oxygen deprivation in the muscle cells of people with back pain. About ten years ago a group of Swedish researchers reported evidence of reduced oxygen levels in the muscles of people with fibromyalgia. (Fibromyalgia is a form of TMS.) In a second paper they reported that blocking the sympathetic nerves (part of the autonomic system) to the painful muscles of patients with fibromyalgia would cause the pain to disappear. The nerve block allowed the blood supply of those muscles to return to normal.

The most recent published study by this group found that painful muscles at the top of the shoulder (trapezius) had less than normal oxygen when exercised. The description of the clinical state of the patients studied suggests that they had TMS.

Because so many of the equivalents of TMS are mediated through the autonomic system, it is logical that TMS is, too. Adding weight to this conclusion is the fact that high blood pressure also comes about through autonomic activity and evidence is accumulating that high blood pressure in many cases is the result of repressed emotions.

If research were to demonstrate some other autonomically induced pain pathology, I would not be disturbed. What's important is not the method the brain uses to produce symptoms; it is the fact that the brain *is* inducing symptoms. I have focused on the oxygen deprivation concept because it is the most logical one available and there is laboratory evidence for it.

Since the mild alteration in oxygen supply may involve muscles, nerves or tendons, a large number of symptoms fall under this diagnosis.

UNIVERSALITY OF MINDBODY DISORDERS

A cruel irony is that the cause of the most common disorders is unrecognized or rejected by the purveyors of medical care. Most of the illnesses that plague us are mindbody in nature. Here are statistics on doctor visits compiled by the National Center for Health Statistics for 1992:

Sore throat	17 million
Backache	14 million
Stomachache	12 million
Headache	10 million

In my experience backache, stomachache and headache are almost always psychologically induced. Upper respiratory infections are heavily influenced by emotional factors, which either reduce or enhance the efficiency of the immune system to resist or overcome infection.

It is important for people to know that emotionally induced physical processes are normal. The reason is clear. We all suffer the stresses and strains of everyday life, particularly if we try to be conscientious and good. "Normal" people are constantly under pressure and always generating unconscious anger-rage.

If you find someone who has never experienced any of these common conditions, you will have found the rare person who has never had a mindbody symptom.

THE WORK OF CANDACE PERT AND COMPANY

A discussion of the theoretical and practical clinical manifestations of the mindbody phenomenon would be incomplete without noting the huge contribution of Candace Pert. It was her suggestion to join the words *mind* and *body*. In my view, she and her colleagues have done the most exciting work in this field. It is particularly important because she is a laboratory scientist, a practitioner of "hard science.".

To my knowledge her research group was the first to speak of the biochemistry of emotions.

Chemicals called neuropeptides have a connection with specific receptors, like a key and a lock. For example, morphine reduces pain because it connects with and activates receptors in the body that reduce pain. Receptors exist for feelings of rage, joy, hunger, pain, pleasure, grief, and for all emotions, as well as for body reactions like appetite, sexual behavior and water balance.

The limbic system in the brain (see Figures 1 and 2) is an important seat of emotions. Two structures in the limbic system, the amygdala and the hypothalamus, are particularly rich in neuropeptide receptors.

According to Dr. Pert, "The striking pattern of neuropeptide distribution in mood-regulating areas of brain, as well as their role in mediating communication throughout the whole organism, makes neuropeptides the obvious candidates for the biochemical mediation of emotion."

Neuropeptides have been found in many locations, like the spleen and the spinal cord. Monocytes, cells of the body's immune system, carry neuropeptide receptors and travel throughout the body.

The study of neuropeptides and their receptors suggests a network in which information of all kinds, including emotional information, is circulated throughout the body, allowing organs and systems to affect each other. The distinction between brain and body is disappearing, since functions that were thought to originate exclusively in the brain are now found elsewhere, and vice versa. Insulin, thought to be produced only in the pancreas, is now known to be made and stored in the brain, and there is a heavy concentration of insulin receptors in the limbic system.

This is magnificent research and there is certain to be more of it. However, we still have the "black box," that mysterious domain that prompts so many questions. How does the brain do what it does? What is the process that allows us to communicate with each other? How do we think? How are emotions elaborated? How does the brain decide to produce a psychosomatic reaction and choose its location?

These questions probably cannot be answered by laboratory science. They may require a new epistemology, that is, a whole new way of thinking about and studying these matters. In the meantime we must get along as best we can, make our observations, test them and use them, even though we can't explain exactly how they work. Benjamin Franklin once said, "Nor is it of much Importance to us to know the Manner in which Nature executes her Laws; 'tis enough to know the Laws themselves."

Keeping Dr. Pert's work in mind, if we look at Figures 1 and 2, we can easily see how an emotion might stimulate a physical disorder through either the autonomic nervous system or alteration of immune function. This is not hypothetical. It happens. It is only difficult to explain at a fundamental level, the level of the "black box."

Let us go on now for a look at these common mindbody disorders.

PART TWO

The Physical Manifestations
of Mindbody Disorders

3

Introduction to the

Tension Myositis Syndrome:

Manifestations in Low Back and Legs

The pain-producing process of TMS may involve three types of tissue: muscle, nerve and tendon. As for muscle, the brain has chosen to target only what are known as postural muscles—the muscles of the neck, shoulders and entire back. Some are involved more frequently than others.

Not illogically, when nerves are involved they are found in and around the muscles chosen for an attack. For example, when lumbar or buttock muscles are the target, the lumbar spinal and/or sciatic nerves may be involved as well. TMS is unpredictable: Sometimes only muscles may be involved; sometimes only nerves.

Any tendon in the body may be a target. Some are more commonly involved than others. With the advent of repetitive stress injuries, we are seeing many more tendon problems.

Low Back and Leg Pain

Statistically, TMS occurs most commonly in the low back; one or both legs may be involved at the same time. The pain may come on suddenly while you are engaging in some physical activity or gradually, without any obvious reason. Often patients report having heard a pop or snap at the moment of onset but we have never found any evidence of a structural derangement that would account for it; it usually occurs when the muscles in the small of the back (lumbar) are the primary ones involved. Although you have done this physical activity many times before, the sudden stab of pain makes you believe the activity is the cause of the pain and that you have been injured. The pain may be in the muscles on one or both sides of the lumbar area and/or lower down, including the upper buttock, occasionally out to the hip area. Lumbar muscle involvement may tilt the trunk to one side.

Lumbar pain may be excruciating, suggesting that the muscles are in spasm, a tight contraction of muscle that will not release. Most people have experienced this with leg cramps, usually in the calf muscle. Leg cramps can be stopped by stretching the muscle involved. Unfortunately, TMS cannot be stopped by stretching, which is why people who have suffered attacks dread a recurrence. Spasms may persist for hours or recur for days and can only be managed with strong painkillers. Back and buttock pain is the result of something happening in muscle. When the spasm has been broken, you may continue to have a dull, burning or pressure pain. Persistent stiffness is part of the same syndrome and may go on for weeks or months.

The lumbar paraspinal and buttock muscles are usually involved in low back and buttock muscle pain. Infrequently, the muscles that form the floor of the pelvis, in the area known as the perineum (between the genital organs in front and the anal opening in back), are the site of TMS. This is usually frightening to the patient and puzzling to the doctor, but is no cause for concern, since it is a classic manifestation of TMS.

Leg pain, usually unilateral but occasionally on both sides, may begin in the buttock and radiate down the outer aspect of the thigh and leg to the foot, or it may go down the back of the thigh, then radiate around to the front of the leg and top of the foot. In some cases the pain radiates to the groin and upper anterior thigh, and very occasionally to the scrotum or vulva. There are many different patterns of involvement: Sometimes the thigh or the entire leg is spared, with pain only in the bottom or the top of the foot.

This great variability in location is characteristic of TMS and is far better explained by TMS than by a structural diagnosis.

In addition to pain in the leg, sensations of numbness or tingling are very common—and frightening. Even more disturbing is the perception of weakness in various parts of the leg. Sometimes we see concrete evidence of reduced muscle strength—buckling at the knee, difficulty elevating the fore part of the foot (foot drop), or difficulty standing on one's toes. These findings are common in TMS and are no cause for concern.

The leg pain may be sharp, dull, aching or burning and is often severe; some patients describe feelings of pressure or stiffness.

While low back and buttock pain is due to muscle involvement, leg symptoms are the result of the inclusion of one or more nerves in the pathological process. Any deviation from the normal in body tissues is called pathological whether it's mild or severe, benign or malignant. In the case of TMS the process is invariably benign, though the symptoms may be exceedingly severe. So widespread, variable and intense is the pain of TMS in some cases that it would seem impossible to attribute it to a structural abnormality, such as a herniated disc. Yet that is commonly done.

The Nerves Involved in Low Back and Leg Pain

Think of the nervous system as an electrical network of a special kind: Wires (nerve fibers) run from the brain, down through the spinal cord, and connect with other wires that go to muscles, bringing messages for movement. These wires are known as motor nerve fibers. What is special about the nervous system, however, is that other nerve fibers run in the opposite direction, from the skin, muscles, joints, tendons, all bringing sensory messages of pain, temperature, position of body parts and many other sensations, back to the brain so that it can know what is going on and what it must do. These are called sensory nerve fibers. The spinal nerves peel off from the spinal cord from the neck down to the sacrum (at the end of the tailbone) and are composed of both motor and sensory nerve fibers, bringing messages to and from the brain.

It is important to know the anatomical relationship between the intervertebral discs of the spine and the spinal nerves that are near them. Discs are interposed between the bodies of spinal bones to act as shock absorbers and facilitate twisting. Therefore, one identifies the location of a disc by the two vertebral bodies it lies between: the lumbar 4–lumbar 5 disc (L4–L5), for example. (There are seven cervical spine bones, twelve thoracic and five lumbar.)

At any given level of the spine, nerves peel off from the spinal cord, one on each side, passing by one of the intervertebral discs. The lumbar 5 spinal nerves pass by the L4–L5 disc. The sacral 1 spinal nerves pass the disc located between the fifth and last vertebral body and the sacrum, the L5–S1 disc.

This anatomical propinquity is a source of much trouble; if the patient has a herniation of the L4–L5 disc and manifests leg pain, the pain will invariably be blamed on the herniation, though in my experience it is rarely responsible. This diagnosis is the basis for a great deal of back surgery.

If the lumbar muscles are the site of TMS involvement, the nerves that may be involved are the lumbar spinal nerves.

For instance, let's say that the lumbar spinal nerve serving the groin, L1, is involved in the TMS process; it is mildly oxygen-deprived. It contains no motor fibers involved with TMS, but the sensory fibers tell the brain what is going on in the groin area. When sensory fibers are oxygen-deprived, a variety of symptoms may ensue, including pain of all kinds, burning or pressure sensations, numbness or tingling. Any of these symptoms in the groin, and occasionally the scrotum or vulva, tell you that the L1 spinal nerve on that side is involved.

L2, L3 or L4 spinal nerves carry important motor fibers to the anterior thigh muscles (the quadriceps). If one or more of these spinal nerves are involved, the tendon reflex at the knee (knee jerk) may be weak or absent. The quadriceps muscle may be weak also. L4 contributes with L5 to the muscles that elevate the foot and toes, which helps to avoid tripping while walking. Weakness of these muscles results in foot drop; partial or complete foot drop is very common in TMS.

Lumbar spinal nerves 2 through 5 provide sensory function to the front and sides of the leg. Pain in the anterior and lateral thigh is often called meralgia paresthetica, a descriptive term, though no one knows its cause. The pain is quite clearly a manifestation of TMS.

If someone has a herniated disc at the lowest level—the L5–S1 disc, which may affect S1, the first sacral spinal nerve—and has pain or other sensory abnormalities involving the front of the leg, one must assume that the disc pathology is not responsible for the pain because S1 serves the back of the leg. Conversely, people with disc herniations at L4–L5—affecting the fifth lumbar spinal nerve, L5—often have pain in the back of the leg, once more proving that the disc pathology is not responsible for the pain, since the back of the leg is supplied by spinal nerves S1 and S2 and *not by*

L5. TMS often involves spinal nerves and is the cause of the pain in these cases.

These diagnostic discrepancies first suggested to me that the herniated disc might not be the cause of the pain. Occasionally the location of the herniation and symptoms will match. This may be more than coincidence, for I have come to believe that the clever brain is aware of the existence of the herniation and chooses to locate the symptoms in the proper area purposely.

Sciatica

Another notorious peripheral nerve is frequently involved in TMS leg pain—the sciatic. The term *sciatica* is familiar to everyone; although doctors and patients use it as a diagnosis, it only refers to pain in the leg. Patients are routinely told a herniated disc is pressing on the sciatic nerve, producing pain. This is an anatomical impossibility. What the medical adviser means is that the herniated disc material is pressing on one of the spinal nerves that sends a branch to the sciatic nerve. Five spinal nerves send branches to the sciatic nerve— L3, L4, L5, S1 and S2. Neurophysiologic logic suggests that although continued compression of a nerve might be painful for a short time, it would soon result in a total loss of feeling because the nerve could not continue to function in the face of persistent compression. In practice, I have found that the lumbar spinal nerves in the small of the back and/or the sciatic nerve itself are frequently implicated in the TMS process and that it is oxygen deprivation, and not nerve compression, that causes the symptoms. That is why people with "sciatica" have pain in so many different parts of the leg, in such different patterns, sometimes shifting from one side to the other. A structural abnormality, like a herniated disc, could not produce such a clinical picture. Many patients with sciatica have no demonstrable structural abnormality on X-ray or imaging studies.

How can I be sure that TMS and not the disc or some other structural abnormality is causing the pain? Over many years I have seen thousands of patients with disc and other structural abnormalities who were told that these changes were responsible for the pain. Their histories and physical examinations suggested the diagnosis of TMS; they were treated accordingly and promptly got better, often after weeks or months of disabling pain.

Pavlovian Conditioning—Programming

One of the most important clinical features of TMS is the tendency for sufferers to develop a specific pattern of pain, including what time of day or night they will have pain, what activities or postures will bring it on, what things they can and cannot do.

These are programmed reactions. They develop automatically and unconsciously by association, just as Pavlov's dogs learned to associate the presentation of food with the sound of a bell. Once the dogs were programmed he had only to ring the bell and they began to salivate. Human beings are just as programmable as animals. Some of these patterns are very common, others are bizarre. For example, it is quite striking that a high proportion of low-back-pain patients cannot sit without having severe pain after only a few minutes. Some can tolerate certain kinds of chairs but not others. Most cannot take sitting in a car, particularly the driver's seat. Another patient with pain in the same location will report that sitting is fine but the pain will begin after being up and around for only a few minutes. Either of these problems can be disruptive to a person's daily life. Someone with pain in the high lumbar area, nowhere near the sitting part of the anatomy, may complain of the same thing.

It has become clear over the years that pattern development, universal in patients with TMS, is the result of Pavlovian conditioning or, to use a more modern word, programming. We very quickly and unconsciously associate these activities, postures and times of the day and night with the onset of pain. Like Pavlov's dogs, who associated the sound of the bell with the presentation of food, we associate various phenomena with the onset of pain.

Some common patterns:

1. You wake up feeling pretty good, but the pain gets worse as the day goes on; by evening you can barely get around.

2. Mornings are the worst; you struggle to get out of bed. A hot shower makes you feel a little better and by the time you leave for work you're able to get around; as the day goes on you feel better and better.

3. You feel pretty good during the day but the nights are terrible; you're in and out of bed all night and can't find a comfortable position; popping pills all night is common.

4. You sleep well at night but the pain during the day is terrible.

5. Every night you wake up at exactly three o'clock with severe pain; you can set your clock by it; it never fails.

6. You have your own truck and can load and unload it all day long without any pain; however, you experience severe pain when you lean over the sink to shave.

7. Standing in one place invariably brings on the pain; it's terrible waiting in line at the supermarket.
8. As soon as you walk onto the tennis court, before you even hit a ball, the pain begins.
9. You windsurf but can't sit on a soft chair.
10. You can only walk a block before the pain begins, but you can play eighteen holes of golf without pain.
11. You're fine on a horse but get pain when climbing stairs.
12. You can hike in the mountains for two hours without pain, but you find walking on concrete very painful.

Here is an excerpt from a letter that describes the programming process beautifully:

> Within two months after going through your program, my symptoms had almost completely disappeared. But much more important was the disappearance of my constant fear of injuring myself. Perhaps the point at which I knew I'd been "cured" was when I found the courage to get on the exercycle which had been gathering dust for years in the corner of my bedroom. In the past, every time I'd tried to use it, even for a minute, my back would bother me for days or weeks afterwards. No chiropractor or orthopedist ever gave me an explanation for this, as I could ride a ten-speed bicycle (when my back wasn't bothering me much) without a problem, even though I was hunched over in the familiar position they warned me to avoid. You taught me that my aversion to the exercycle was a conditioned response, that I believed I had injured myself on the bike once upon a time and anticipated further injury if I tried it again.

After a few weeks of going through the daily reminders and stealing glances at the culprit machine out of the corner of my eye, I was ready. The first time I tried it, even though I cycled for only five minutes, I knew the nightmare was over. By that time, I was pretty well convinced that nothing would happen to me, and all I had to do was try it. Of course, that was exactly right. I quickly built up my time and speed on the machine; I admit that I was so taken by this new-found freedom that I became a bit fanatical about using it for a while.

Fear, misinformation and disability dominate our beliefs about back pain to such an extent that it is no wonder we become programmed to develop pain in association with a wide variety of phenomena. When and how the programming takes place is unclear except that it happens very soon after the pain begins. Programming is a real and very important part of the clinical picture and should be a source of reassurance to people with back pain because the pattern of pain is the product of conditioning—not a pathological condition. In other words, sitting doesn't bring on pain because sitting is bad for the back. The pain begins when it does because the onset of pain is programmed. Fortunately, that programming is reversible. My patients become deconditioned a few weeks after they begin the treatment program. People who get better by studying my books on TMS are deconditioned by the knowledge acquired from the books.

Physical Examination for Patients with Low Back and Leg Pain

The examination begins by observing how the patient walks and stands. Weakness in a leg is not uncommon, so the patient may favor one leg. Occasionally weakness in the muscles that elevate the foot is severe enough that it can be detected during the gait cycle. Tilting of the trunk to one side or the other is common when the lumbar paraspinal muscles have been the major site of activity. Asking the patient to bend at the waist is always revealing: Many patients are reluctant to do so because they fear the pain may ensue or because they have been told that bending is bad for the back. Of those who are willing to bend, most will report that they are no longer as flexible as they were. Although some bend normally, without fear or pain, most will complain of back or leg pain when they bend.

Functional testing of ankle and knee muscle strength is done while the patient is upright. Knee and ankle tendon reflexes are tested in the sitting position and give information about motor weakness in the leg.

On the examining table, circulation in the legs is tested by finding the pulses in the foot and ankle. One looks for pain on palpation of tendons around the knees and along the iliotibial band, the long tendon that traverses the entire length of the lateral thigh and passes behind the bony prominence at the hip known as the trochanter. Pain in this tendon is found in about 80 percent of patients with TMS regardless of the site of the pain (neck, shoulders, upper back, midback or low back). The so-called straight leg raising test is done only to see what the patient can do and whether pain is elicited. I find it to be of no diagnostic value.

In the prone position the entire back is palpated for what are called tender points. It has been found that in 99 percent of patients with TMS there is pain on palpation of varying degrees on both sides (bilateral) of the lateral upper buttock, deep in the lumbar paraspinal muscles and the upper trapezius muscles (the top of the shoulders). Once more, this is so regardless of the major site of pain. This suggests very strongly that the process responsible for the pain originates in the central nervous system, in the brain.

Finally, additional neurological tests are done to determine whether any nerve structures have been involved. Finding objective nerve abnormalities does not establish the diagnosis; it permits the physician to discuss and reassure the patient about his or her symptoms.

Conventional Diagnoses for Low Back and Leg Pain

One must bear in mind that any structural abnormality is routinely said to be the cause of pain when found on X-ray or imaging studies in patients with TMS. In my experience they are rarely the source of the pain.

Diagnoses fall into two major categories:

1. Structural abnormalities of the spine, both acquired and congenital
2. Painful muscle disorders of unknown cause

Structural Abnormalities

DEGENERATIVE OSTEOARTHRITIS

Of the structural group, changes in the spine associated with aging are the most common. They are referred to as arthrosis or degenerative osteoarthritis of the spine. They begin as early as the second decade of life and are usually more advanced in those parts of the spine that see the most activity—the last two lumbar vertebrae and the middle of the neck. This group includes osteophyte (spur) formation anywhere in the spine, technically known as spondylosis. Aging changes in the joints of the spine, identified as the facet syndrome, are now thought to be without symptoms, although they were treated as a clinical entity for years.

In 1976, doctors at Hadassah Hospital in Jerusalem reported finding no difference in the incidence of low back pain in people with and without osteoarthritis of the spine.

A group of physicians from the University of Copenhagen compared the X rays of 238 patients with low back pain with those of 66 patients with no history of such pain. They reported no difference in the X rays of the two groups with respect to degeneration of the discs and the presence of spondylosis (bone spurs). They observed that the incidence of these changes increased with age, as might be expected, since they are normal abnormalities.

SPINAL STENOSIS

One of the most important age-related changes is spinal stenosis because it is frequently treated surgically. As we age, the lumbar spinal canal, the space that allows for the passage of the spinal cord or spinal nerves, gradually becomes narrower because of the accumulation of bone spurs. If this condition is found in the TMS patient with severe pain, surgery is recommended and, if the patient is desperate, often performed. Of the large number of patients I have seen with this diagnosis I can recall only one who needed surgery. More convincing is the fact that when these patients are treated for TMS they become pain-free despite the continuing presence of stenosis.

H. L. Rosomoff, a neurosurgeon, has reported that most cases of spinal stenosis can be treated nonsurgically. This is particularly noteworthy, for he treated patients with surgery for many years.

In the first follow-up survey conducted with our patient population, the highest incidence of back pain was between the ages of thirty and sixty. Beyond the age of sixty the incidence dropped considerably. If aging changes were responsible for back pain, one would expect an increase in the incidence with age. Instead, people in the middle years of life, the years of the greatest stress and strain, had these pain syndromes most frequently, strongly suggesting that TMS, and not structural changes in the spine, was the cause of the pain.

INTERVERTEBRAL DISC PATHOLOGY

Statistically, one of the most common and far and away the most troublesome of the aging changes involves the intervertebral discs. They are designed to be intervertebral shock absorbers but begin to wear out at a very early age. The disc between the last lumbar vertebra, L5, and the sacrum is degenerated in most people by the age of twenty. Degeneration means that the disc may lose substance and become narrower, bringing the two vertebral bodies closer together, or disc material may escape through the worn-out enclosing tissue, called annulus fibrosis, with—in order of increasing severity—a resultant bulge or protrusion or extrusion of disc material (nucleus pulposus). Protrusion and extrusion are commonly known as a herniated disc.

It has been my experience that even large extrusions are usually not responsible for continuing pain, though they may cause some pain when they first occur.

For a long time I was disturbed by the fact that the location of the pain in someone with a lumbar disc herniation sometimes correlated accurately with the location of the herniation. For example, if there was a herniation in the vicinity of the first sacral spinal nerve (S1), the pain might be found in the part of the leg served by that nerve. It was easy to see why someone would attribute the patient's pain to the herniation. However, the persistence of symptoms for weeks and months, and the presence of the signs and symptoms of TMS, made it clear that while the disc pathology may have caused some initial pain, *it was not responsible for continuing pain.*

Why would the brain choose to suggest that the disc was the culprit? The answer is to be found in a study of the strategy the brain uses when it creates TMS. It will often initiate symptoms while the person is engaged in some physical activity, the more vigorous the better, to foster the idea that the activity caused the pain. In reality, the physical incident is a trigger for, rather than the cause of, the pain. That is an extremely important concept, for failure to recognize it has kept millions of people in bondage to pain and in fear of physical activity.

Disc herniation, like a physical incident, is a trigger for TMS, and a very clever one at that. The brain is aware of the presence of the disc abnormality and so chooses to locate symptoms in the appropriate place. Often, however, it overshoots and involves too much of the leg, for example, or shifts the pain from one side to the other. In some cases the pain is on the wrong side to begin with.

If this idea seems weird, diabolical or fanciful, remember the purpose of the pain syndrome. It is an illogical reaction of the unconscious mind in response to something that is considered far more dangerous than the pain.

What does the medical literature say about the lumbar herniated discs? Following is a small sample.

H. L. Rosomoff, a neurosurgeon, has found that lumbar disc herniations are responsible for low back and leg pain in fewer than 3 percent of cases and treats his patients conservatively—that is to say, nonsurgically.

Alf Nachemson, a world-renowned student of low back pain, has stated that the cause is unknown in the majority of cases and that patients should be treated conservatively in 98 percent of them.

One research group reported finding lumbar herniated discs on myelography in 108 patients with no back pain. They kept track of them, however, and found that within three years 64 percent of patients had developed nerve symptoms, and researchers concluded that the symptoms were due to the original herniation.

I very much doubt this and suggest that these patients had developed TMS. The idea of late symptomatology is contradicted by a study done by a group of doctors from the Universities of Rome and L'Aquila, who reported that 63 percent of a group of patients with MRI-documented lumbar herniated discs, treated nonsurgically, showed reduction in the size of the herniations when MRIs were repeated six to fifteen months later.

A group from George Washington University reported an interesting study in the journal *Spine* in 1984. Lumbar CT scans on patients without low back pain were reviewed by neuroradiologists who had no knowledge of the patients' clinical histories. They found disc abnormalities, stenosis and other aging changes in 35.4 percent of the entire group of fifty-two people and in 50 percent of the group over forty years of age. These are normal abnormalities, and in most cases do not cause any pain at all.

Richard Deyo, John Loeser and Stanley Bigos from the University of Washington wrote that only 5 to 10 percent of patients with lumbar herniated discs needed surgery, but thought surgery would be necessary if the herniation was documented by CT scan or MRI, was accompanied by typical pain and neurological weakness and failed to respond to six weeks of conservative treatment.

I have found that these criteria for surgery are not dependable, for TMS can produce "typical" pain and neurological changes, and will persist for weeks or months if it is not properly diagnosed and treated.

A more recent study, one that received a great deal of attention in the press, was reported in the *New England Journal of Medicine* by Maureen Jensen and her colleagues. Lumbar

MRIs were done on ninety-eight people with no history of low back or leg pain. Thirty-six percent had normal discs at all levels, 52 percent had a bulging disc at one or more levels, 27 percent had a disc protrusion and 1 percent had an extrusion. Their conclusion: "The discovery by MRI of bulges or protrusions in people with low back pain may frequently be coincidental."

In 1987 I did a follow-up survey on 109 patients with back pain attributed to a herniated disc. The herniation was documented in each case by a CT scan. These patients were treated from 1984 to 1986, before the advent of the MRI. However, the herniation could be accurately ascertained with a CT scan. Each patient was diagnosed with TMS based on history and physical examination, implying that the herniation was not the cause of the pain. They all participated in the educational program, and when interviewed one to three years after treatment, 96 (88 percent) were either completely or sufficiently free of pain to be leading normal lives with no physical restrictions or fears. Eleven (10 percent) were improved but still restricted or fearful to some extent. Two people (2 percent) failed to improve.

During the years that those patients were treated, I made no effort to determine whether prospective patients were receptive to the idea that their pain was emotionally induced, meaning that some patients could not fully accept the diagnosis. Patients who cannot acknowledge psychological causation do not get better. I now screen patients before admitting them to our program.

Medical research appropriately seeks proof of diagnostic theories and new modes of treatment. The best proof of the accuracy of the TMS diagnosis is that we have now reached the point where over 90 percent of our treated patients (often after years of recurrent, disabling pain) become permanently pain-free. I cannot imagine more compelling proof that TMS is the correct diagnosis. The critical factor, with this or any other epidemic, is diagnosis. As long as the medical community continues to reject the diagnosis of TMS, the epidemic will continue.

Other structural diagnoses must be mentioned, since they are routinely blamed for back pain.

SCOLIOSIS

This is a well-known abnormality of the spine in which there is a side-to-side curvature, usually involving most of the spine. Its cause has never been determined. It usually begins in the second decade of life and is invariably painless in teenagers, though the curve may be severe enough to warrant surgery, particularly if it continues to get worse. I find it a source of wonderment that scoliosis in adults is assumed to be painful. Because the doctors don't have an alternative explanation for the pain, logic takes flight. Over and over the pain of TMS is attributed to some structural abnormality or a physical or mechanical process because the medical profession is not aware of the existence of TMS.

I recall a woman who had two surgical procedures for back pain assumed to be caused by scoliosis and was in the hospital for a third. Before her operation, she was discovered by a psychologist on staff who knew about TMS and suggested to the surgeon that there might be a psychological basis for her pain. Instead of undergoing surgery, the woman entered our program. Within a matter of weeks she was free of pain and has remained so.

SPONDYLOLISTHESIS

This is a dramatic-looking abnormality in which a lumbar vertebra has moved out of line with the one below, usually forward. Cases range from mild to severe. The cause of the condition is mysterious, but in my experience the disorder is painless. I have photographs of serial X rays on a young woman who was unaware that she had developed this abnormality because she had no pain. The X rays were done for some other reason and the spondylolisthesis was discovered by accident. This does not surprise me, for I have yet to see someone with spondylolisthesis who did not have TMS.

THE PYRIFORMIS SYNDROME

Deep in the buttock there is a muscle, the pyriformis, which is in close proximity to the sciatic nerve as it passes through the greater sciatic notch on its way into the leg. I do not know where or when the diagnosis was first proposed, but it was theorized that buttock pain was the result of compression of the sciatic nerve by the pyriformis muscle. It has not been scientifically explained why this happens or under what circumstances. In my view the diagnosis is without substance and has only been proposed in the absence of a better explanation for buttock pain. Clearly, TMS provides the best explanation for such pain. The diagnosis of pyriformis syndrome is a fad that appears to be fading away.

OSTEOARTHRITIS OF THE HIP

Another important addition to the list of structural abnormalities wrongfully accused of causing back pain is the arthritic hip. Degenerative changes in the hip joint are fairly common and so is TMS pain in the buttock. Following the usual pattern, the pain is often blamed on the hip joint and hip replacement surgery is done even when the degeneration is relatively mild. I have intervened in some cases before surgery was done and successfully treated the pain nonsurgically. Moreover, I have seen others who had surgery and continued to have pain.

Congenital Abnormalities

Three congenital spinal abnormalities are said to cause back pain: spina bifida occulta, spondylolysis and transitional vertebra. In the first two a piece of bone is missing from the spine, and in the third there is an extra bone. Investigators Alexander Magora and Armin Schwartz found that these abnormalities were just as common in people without back pain as in those with pain. In my experience they do not cause back pain.

Other Diagnoses

FIBROMYALGIA

The ailment that is currently called fibromyalgia (FMS) is a classic manifestation of TMS. The term is one of many designations for a painful disorder that has been known since 1904, when it was first described by Sir William Gowers. Here is a partial list of what it, or conditions like it, have been called through the years: fibrositis, fibromyositis, myofibrositis, myofascial pain, muscular rheumatism, tension myalgia, myalgia, rheumatic myositis, myelogelosis.

Following are diagnostic criteria for fibromyalgia set forth by the American College of Rheumatology:

1. History of widespread pain. The official definition then lists specific parts of the body, covering virtually the entire trunk, front and back, and parts of the arms and legs.
2. Pain in eleven of eighteen tender point sites with finger pressure. The sites are both sides (bilateral) of the following nine locations:
   a. Occiput (the base of the skull)
   b. Low cervical (the back of the neck)

   c. Trapezius muscle (the top of the shoulder)
   d. Supraspinatus muscle (upper back near the shoulder blade)
   e. Second rib (near the middle of the chest in front)
   f. Lateral epicondyle (the elbow region)
   g. Gluteal (the upper, outer part of the buttock)
   h. Greater trochanter (behind the prominent hip bone)
   i. Knee (the inner aspect)

It is not a coincidence that I have found bilateral tender points on finger pressure at three of the nine locations in 98 percent of all patients diagnosed with TMS, regardless of the location of their pain. For example, the patient may complain of pain in the neck and shoulder on one side but will have pain on pressure over the gluteal and hip bone areas as well as the top of the shoulder. Though not as uniformly consistent as those three, many of my patients also have pain on pressure over the elbow, the knee, the base of the skull and the back of the neck.

The painful structures at four of the nine locations—the base of the skull, the hip area, the elbow and the knee—are tendons; involvement of tendons is a prime feature of TMS.

I have maintained for years that fibromyalgia was a severe form of TMS. The similarity of my findings to the diagnostic criteria of the American College of Rheumatology reinforces that diagnostic conclusion.

People with fibromyalgia commonly have psychological symptoms as well. They are often anxious and depressed, have sleep problems and suffer from lack of energy.

Since fibromyalgia is part of TMS, I have seen and successfully treated many patients who had been given that diagnosis before they came to me. Most of my cases did not fulfill the diagnostic criteria set forth by the American College of Rheumatology, but were told they had fibromyalgia nevertheless.

The female/male incidence ratio of fibromyalgia in the United States is ten to one. There are millions of American women languishing with this diagnosis, for they have been told by their medical advisers that the cause of fibromyalgia is unknown and that they must learn to live with the pain. One such patient chose assisted suicide recently.

Clinicians have asked, Is fibromyalgia a separate entity? Only as part of TMS and, therefore, it is a mindbody process. That, of course, explains why it has remained a diagnostic enigma to doctors.

Let us now look at the other disorders in the group.

MYOFASCIAL PAIN SYNDROME AND TEMPEROMANDIBULAR JOINT SYNDROME

Fibromyalgia, myofascial pain syndrome (MPS) and temperomandibular joint syndrome (TMJ) are often discussed together in the medical literature. I believe they are different manifestations of TMS. They vary in anatomy, epidemiology, clinical pattern and severity. Contrasting fibromyalgia and MPS is interesting and illustrative. The gender ratio is ten to one female for fibromyalgia and two to one male for MPS. Fibromyalgia produces tender points all over: the front and back of the trunk, the legs and arms. In MPS they are localized in the back. Fibromyalgia patients are stiff, tired and usually anxious, depressed, insomniac. This is generally not true of people with MPS. The person with fibromyalgia seldom gets better.

What they have in common are pain, the same mild oxygen deprivation and, at a very deep level, a similar psychological profile—that is, repressed rage.

The TMJ syndrome produces pain in the muscles of the

jaw that most dentists attribute to abnormalities in the temporomandibular (jaw) joint. I have found that what is going on in the jaw muscles is similar to the TMS process in the back. Joint abnormalities are the result rather than the cause of the symptoms.

The site of pain is muscle.

I have given only a cursory description of these disorders, for it is beyond the scope and purpose of this book to review them exhaustively. What must be stated unequivocally is that they are psychogenic, induced by unconscious emotional phenomena. Fibromyalgia, MPS, and TMJ are part of TMS. The multitude of studies that have been done around the world to understand them can only identify the details or consequences of the processes, not their cause. Thus far, no one has mounted studies to test the hypothesis that they are psychogenic, though some have flirted with the idea. Until such studies are done, doctors will continue to flounder. The consistent success we have had in treating TMS, even when it was originally diagnosed as fibromyalgia, MPS or TMJ, should point the way.

REFLEX SYMPATHETIC DYSTROPHY

This malady is characterized by pain, swelling, tight and shiny skin and bone abnormalities that can be seen on X ray. It may involve one or more limbs and tends to be extremely disabling. The symptoms and physical findings on examination are said to be caused by excessive discharge of sympathetic nerves resulting in widespread reduction in blood flow and oxygen deprivation. It is similar to what happens with TMS but is more severe and involves muscles, nerves, tendons, skin and bone.

The following case history is illustrative.

A twenty-eight-year-old woman began to have pain in both shoulders and arms during the sixth month of her pregnancy. By the time the baby was born the pain had become much worse and she was severely disabled. The working diagnosis was reflex sympathetic dystrophy, for which she received the standard treatment of physical therapy and steroids, with no improvement. During the first year after her diagnosis she was in psychotherapy for brief periods on two occasions, to no avail. She attended a pain center seven months just prior to her consultation with me with no apparent benefit.

When I first saw her she complained of severe pain in the shoulders, arms and upper back. She also complained of severe weakness in the shoulders and arms, and weakness, soreness and stiffness in the low back, buttock and knees. She could tolerate even the mildest of physical activity for only thirty minutes, after which she had to rest for thirty to forty-five minutes. Clearly, she was unable to function as mother and homemaker. As a teenager she had had a small intestine disorder, asthma and hay fever.

The neurological examination was normal. The range of motion was limited in both shoulders; there was pain on finger pressure on top of both shoulders, the outer aspect of both buttocks and the sides of both thighs (the iliotibial bands).

Her history and physical examination suggested two diagnoses: TMS and psychogenic regional pain (see Chapter 2).

She participated in our teaching program and immediately began group and individual psychotherapy. She grasped the diagnostic concepts quickly, but progress in psychotherapy was slow. However, eight months after beginning work with our team she began to care for her baby to a limited degree. Twelve months into the program she was able to tolerate being up for five hours at a time, and at sixteen months she was functional for half the day. She continued to improve slowly but steadily, eventually becoming a full-time mother and homemaker. Moreover, she resumed tennis and skiing and, demonstrating complete psychological and physical recovery, was ready to have her second child.

This outcome would not have been possible without the correct diagnosis and effective psychotherapy, both of which were crucial. Her symptoms were clearly psychogenic. Powerful emotional factors can induce pathological discharges of sympathetic nerves.

POST-POLIO SYNDROME

In recent years something called the post-polio syndrome has received a lot of attention. It refers to people with residual leg weakness from childhood poliomyelitis who experience increasing weakness as they get older, along with pain in the buttock and legs. Increasing weakness was medically documented years ago as a common occurrence in people who had poliomyelitis. The pain is a new phenomenon, hence the creation of a new syndrome. In the patients I have seen with this problem the pain is due to TMS, no doubt engendered by the fear and frustration associated with increasing weakness. The pain is not part of the poliomyelitis.

Here is another example of failure to recognize the presence of TMS and the creation of a new clinical entity as a consequence. Thirty years ago I worked with many post-polio patients who were suffering the distressing experience of increasing weakness. TMS was not in vogue then as it is now and they had no accompanying pain—so there was no post-polio syndrome. I tried to help them adjust to their loss of strength, sometimes with assistive devices, but always with a lot of support and advice.

TENSION MYALGIA

This diagnosis has been made at the Mayo Clinic for close to fifty years. It refers to pain in muscles (myalgia).

Since the word *tension* is used here to refer to psychological rather than muscle tension, this would seem to be a very enlightened diagnosis. However, the following excerpt from a paper published in the *Mayo Clinic Proceedings* by Jeffrey Thompson is revealing (italics mine):

"The word tension suggests that psychologic tension or stress may play a role. When the diagnosis is presented in this way, patients are more willing to accept the possibility of psychologic influences on their muscle pain disorder and are more likely to take the necessary steps to address them. At the same time, the physician is acknowledging that a *psychologic disturbance is not the primary cause.*"

The statement may sound contradictory but it is not. The doctor is saying that psychological factors are aggravating the pain, not causing it, which goes to the heart of the pain epidemic in which the United States is now engulfed. In fibromyalgia, tension myalgia and other similar diagnostic entities, contemporary medicine may admit that psychological factors are playing a "major role" but it cannot accept the idea that they are the primary cause. In essence, they are left without a diagnosis since psychology, in their view, is only aggravating the problem.

Another interesting point: The author states, "Presented in this way patients are more willing to accept the possibility of psychologic influences on the muscle pain disorder and are more likely to take the necessary steps to address them."

Taking steps to address psychological factors would only eliminate that portion of the pain that was worsened by psychological factors. The underlying pain would continue, for they would not have addressed the cause.

I must confess to feeling great sadness at the utter confusion and inability of medicine to deal with these pain problems. They are wedded to the idea that "a psychologic disturbance is not the primary cause." Indeed, it is not a psychologic disturbance; it is our normal state. We are all programmed to react to inner tensions with physical symptoms. Failure to recognize that fact breeds epidemics.

Conventional Treatment of Low Back and Leg Pain

Treatment varies to some degree depending on the structural diagnosis. For example, if the diagnosis of herniated disc is made based on CT scan or MRI findings and if the patient's pain is severe, surgery is often recommended even if there are no neurological changes in the leg. If neurological changes are present, surgery will almost certainly be offered. The same thing is true when the pain is attributed to the other structural diagnoses just described.

One man wrote, "My foot-drop went away, as you said it would, despite the fact that I had been advised to have surgery by two prominent surgeons." Another wrote, "I was told you can't run away from it [back and leg pain], you must have surgery. Well, I didn't run away; I sat instead through two of your lectures and have been free of pain ever since" [seven years at the time of this writing].

If surgery is not recommended for patients with severe pain, the prescription will be bed rest and, almost inevitably, an anti-inflammatory medication, either nonsteroidal or a steroid (cortisone-type drug). The latter may be administered as an epidural (base of the spine) injection. If after two or three weeks in bed the pain persists, physical therapy is usually prescribed and may continue for weeks or months.

What are these patients like three or four months later? The pain has continued; they are worried, upset, fearful, unable to engage in their usual physical activities and on the verge of depression. They often consult different conventional physicians like orthopedists, neurologists, physiatrists, rheumatologists or specialists in sports medicine, to no avail.

Now they begin to try what mainstream medicine calls unconventional medicine and what others have identified as holistic or alternative medicine. This means seeing a chiropractor, osteopath, acupuncturist, massage therapist, nutritionist, naturopath, exercise specialist and so on. They may be helpful, but some pain persists and the admonition to beware of physical activity like running, sports or weight lifting means that the patients remain unhappy and concerned and partially disabled.

Regardless of the conventional diagnosis, people with recurrent low back and leg pain are usually fearful and disabled in various ways. Fearing pain, they are afraid they will injure themselves, and so avoid many physical activities. Careful of their movements, they often use lumbar corsets and special pillows for sitting or in bed. They are afraid to bend, lift, cross their legs, lie on their stomachs or swim the crawl or breast stroke because they have been taught that arching the back causes pain. They are told that a short leg and flat feet cause back pain, as do weak abdominal muscles. They are told that strong stomach muscles protect you from pain and that running is bad for the spine. (If that were true, how could *Homo sapiens* have survived the thousands of years living in the wild?) They believe that a hard mattress is best for sleeping. Their lives are dominated by their backs; pain is often the last thing they are aware of before they fall asleep at night and the first thing they think of upon awakening. They are drowning in a sea of misinformation.

It is striking how often patients will report that they have tried every conceivable treatment and spent a lot of money in the process. Many tell me candidly that they see me because nothing else has worked. I tend to see the most persistent cases, people who have had recurrent episodes for ten, twenty and thirty years. Perhaps once a month I may see a patient who has not first visited another doctor; however, for most patients the history will invariably be one of recurrent pain episodes for many years and disenchantment with all the treatments that have been tried.

Medicine is slowly acknowledging that psychosocial factors play a role in the back pain epidemic that currently afflicts the industrialized world. A study published in the journal *Spine* in 1991 by Stanley Bigos and a large group of collaborators at the University of Washington identified psychological factors as more important than physical ones in predicting who would report an industrial back injury.

In Finland a large group of investigators found that back pain patients who were advised to continue their usual activities, as opposed to taking bed rest for two days or doing "back-mobilizing exercises," had a statistically better outcome in duration of pain, pain intensity, bending the back and ability to work.

Traditional medicine still has no awareness of the nature of the mindbody process that initiates back pain, but perhaps these studies on the fringe of psychology will engender a more open attitude.

4

Manifestations in Upper Back, Neck, Shoulders and Arms

Somewhere between 60 and 65 percent of people with TMS have symptoms in the low back and/or legs. Most of them acknowledge having had neck and shoulder symptoms of varying severity currently or sometime in the past. This is no surprise, since the neck and top of the shoulder are the second most common location for TMS; it is the major site of pain in 20 to 25 percent of the TMS population. TMS can involve many different locations in the entire back; it tends to move around even during the course of an episode. However, the brain apparently needs to create only one major site at a time, so if it's not in the low back it may be in the neck and shoulder.

The most frequently involved muscle in this area is the upper trapezius, which extends from the back of the head down to the top of the shoulder and out to the bony prominence that can be felt over the shoulder, one on either side, of course. All or part of the upper trapezius muscle may be painful. As with low back pain, people often report doing something strenuous just before the onset of pain. In many cases it comes on slowly or is there when the person wakes up in the morning. It can be as disabling as low back pain, particularly if there are symptoms in the arm and hand. When the pain is relatively mild, patients report that the muscles feel tense. People tend to associate sensations in the neck area with nervous tension. They rarely do so with low back pain.

Other muscles near the shoulder blades may be involved, but much less frequently than the upper trapezius.

Cervical Nerve Involvement

As in low back, pain may radiate into the arm and hand, along with feelings of numbness, tingling and weakness. Tendon reflexes may be reduced or absent and there can be measurable muscle weakness. The nerve structures responsible for these symptoms are the cervical spinal nerves and/or the brachial plexus, which receives branches from cervical spinal nerves C5, C6, C7 and C8 and thoracic spinal nerve T1. The brachial plexus then divides into all the peripheral nerves serving the arm and hand, such as the radial, median and ulnar. This important collection of nerves (plexus) is located deep in the area below the upper trapezius muscle. It cannot be reached by pressing on the upper trapezius muscle but is frequently involved when TMS is active in that muscle, meaning that parts of the plexus will be mildly oxygen-deprived. It is characteristic of TMS that when a large nerve structure like the sciatic nerve or the brachial plexus is involved, only parts of it are affected. That is why sciatica is not a single-symptom description. Many different parts of the leg—the front, the back, the sides—may hurt. The pain may move around, affecting the thigh but missing the leg; it may involve only the top or bottom of the foot. The same is true of the brachial plexus, so that sometimes there is pain only around the shoulder and top of the arm, or different parts of the arm and hand. I have seen every variety imaginable. This would not be true if the cause of the pain were a structural disorder.

On rare occasions I have seen weakness of the muscle that holds the scapula (shoulder blade) in place, so that the scapula tends to protrude (winging). This muscle is served by the long thoracic nerve of Bell, which receives branches from cervical spinal nerves C5 and C6. TMS may involve either the spinal nerves or the long thoracic nerve.

TMS and Cranial Nerves

Two mysterious disorders have plagued diagnosticians for years. They are known as Bell's palsy and trigeminal neuralgia and involve two of the twelve so-called cranial nerves. They arise in the brain stem, the section of the central nervous system below the brain and above the spinal cord, and serve the head and its specialized organs, the eyes, ears, mouth and throat. They bring movement instructions from the brain, carrying back sensory information and providing the special organs with a link to the brain.

The fifth cranial nerve (trigeminal) is a pure sensory nerve, bringing sensation to the face and teeth. For years it has been recognized as the source of excruciating facial and dental pain; the condition is called trigeminal neuralgia, or tic douloureux. No one has ever been able to explain it.

A number of years ago I had an episode of dental nerve pain that could not be explained. After suffering it for a few months, I was looking at anatomical drawings of the nervous system with patients one day when I came upon a particularly vivid depiction of the nerve supply to the teeth, branches of the fifth nerve, and immediately wondered if the dental pain might be TMS of the trigeminal nerve. I concluded that it was—and the pain was gone in less than forty-eight hours. This is an example of the therapeutic power of awareness, as will be described in Part III of this book.

Since I am known as a back specialist, I am not generally consulted by people with facial pain. However, circumstances recently brought such a case to my attention. Fortunately for the patient, his history was extremely suggestive.

He was in the midst of divorce proceedings that had taken a nasty turn. This was particularly upsetting to him as he hated and sedulously avoided conflict. During the proceedings his facial pain began.

Earlier in this section I discussed how people with TMS become programmed and may have symptoms at strange times. This man had facial pain when he lay in certain positions or was engaged in activities that could have had nothing to do with the function of the fifth nerve.

Luckily, he was open to the suggestion that the highly unpleasant events had enraged him internally and were the source of his pain. The pain promptly disappeared.

A series of two cases is not impressive, nor is it conclusive proof of the psychogenic cause of these disorders. One day we may have the research tools to demonstrate the local oxygen deprivation to the fifth and seventh nerve that is probably the basis for these mysterious disorders.

The seventh cranial nerve, in contrast to the fifth, is a pure motor nerve, serving the muscles of the face (one on each side). Dysfunction of this nerve causes the distinctive appearance of someone with Bell's palsy, with loss of forehead wrinkles, failure of the eyelid to close and drooping of the face and lips on the affected side.

I have never seen a patient with Bell's palsy, but Graeme Taylor's monumental book on psychosomatic medicine contains a wonderful case history. One of Dr. Taylor's patients developed Bell's palsy when Dr. Taylor discontinued psychotherapy. I believe the patient was unconsciously enraged at having been abandoned and, like someone with TMS, developed a physical disorder to prevent her rage from becoming conscious. Bell's palsy is very likely the result of oxygen deprivation of the seventh cranial nerve. (This case is discussed further in the appendix.)

Conventional Diagnoses

Osteoarthritis and "Pinched Nerve"

When the pain is restricted to the muscles of the neck and shoulder it may be attributed to a strain. If there are arm or hand symptoms, X rays, CT scans or MRIs invariably show a structural abnormality. Bone spurs (osteophytes) are common, and may narrow the openings through which spinal nerves emerge (intervertebral foramina). However, one of these openings would have to be virtually obliterated before causing any problem with the emerging nerve. Despite that, doctors continue to claim that the nerve is "pinched" and attribute the arm and hand pain to that. As with the low back and leg, one can often find neurologic changes on physical examination that do not correlate anatomically with the location of the bone spur. As in the leg, the symptoms are due to TMS and not the spur.

Once more the medical literature supports the observation that structural abnormalities are rarely the cause of pain. A study published by research workers from the Medical College of Wisconsin in 1986 demonstrated that degenerative changes (osteoarthritis) in the neck, including spur formation, narrowing of the disc space and bone thickening (end plate) sclerosis, were common, particularly as one got older, and very often resulting in no pain.

In my experience, TMS, not structural abnormalities, is responsible for the pain in most cases.

Whiplash

Another problem in this area is known as whiplash injury. The usual scenario is that your car is hit from behind, your head bounces back, and sometime in the ensuing hours or days your neck begins to hurt. This often develops into a full-blown episode with pain in one or both arms, down the back, even to the low back, and weeks or months of treatment. X rays are normal, there is no structural damage, and any sprain or strain involved should heal in a few weeks at the most. Symptoms persist because the brain has taken the opportunity of the minor accident to initiate TMS.

Here is a situation I see over and over with TMS: Physical incidents, like the hit-from-behind accident, a slip or a fall, doing physical work, engaging in a sport, and repetitive work motions are used by the brain as excuses to start up TMS. They are triggers, not causes, and must be identified as such. We have incredible healing mechanisms that have evolved over millions of years. No matter how severe, injuries heal. Continuing pain is always the signal that TMS has begun. Consider that a fracture of the largest bone in the body, the femur (thigh bone), takes only six weeks to heal and will be stronger at the fracture site than it was before the break.

Strong support that whiplash is part of TMS came to my attention in the Medical Science section of the *New York Times* from a piece published in the May 7, 1996, issue titled "In One Country, Chronic Whiplash Is Uncompensated (and Unknown)."

Quoting an article from the British medical journal *Lancet*, the reporter noted that whiplash was unheard of in Lithuania, while in Norway it was of epidemic proportions. Dr. Harald Schrader, a neurologist at University Hospital in Trondheim and the apparent leader of the research team, was quoted as saying that there was "an explosion of chronic whiplash cases in Norway," that there are "70,000 cases in a country of 4.2 million people who feel they have chronic disability because of whiplash." At one point he said, "It's mass hysteria." Dr. Schrader and his team went to Lithuania and documented the fact that whiplash was unknown in that country.

This is confirmation of the psychogenic nature of whiplash. Since the Norwegian doctors are unaware of the existence of TMS, they conclude that patients are motivated by the desire to be compensated for injury, though there may be no injury. This is known as secondary gain. What confounds the situation is that these patients have real pain; they are not faking it to get money. What they have is TMS. But neither they nor their doctors know the true nature of the process, so the doctors think the patients are lying or exaggerating, and the patients are indignant at the suggestion. The *Times* article said that when the findings of the study were publicized in Norway, the leader of the whiplash patients' organization threatened to sue the doctor who led the study. Little wonder.

This report also illustrates the "social contagion" at work with psychosomatic disorders. People will unconsciously choose symptoms that are in vogue and considered legitimate physical disorders by their doctors, which is why the syndromes of neck and back pain are of epidemic proportions in most of the Western world today.

This is a daunting public health problem, for neither the medical profession nor the patients know the nature of the disorder. Until authoritative medicine considers the idea that emotions induce physical symptoms, this health problem will persist.

Cervical Herniated Disc

As in the low back, one of the most common diagnoses in the cervical area is herniated disc. Despite the greater proximity of the herniated disc material to the spinal cord in the neck, evidence is accumulating that such herniations may not be dangerous and can be treated conservatively (nonsurgical).

This is good news, for my work indicates that, as in the low back, the herniation is not responsible for the pain or neurological symptoms in the arms—that TMS is the culprit.

For over forty years evidence has shown that structural abnormalities in the cervical spine region rarely cause symptoms. Donald McRae, of the Montreal Neurological Institute, published a paper in 1956 in which he said that anyone over thirty years of age may have herniation of a disc in the neck without symptoms.

Nineteen years later, Allan Fox and his colleagues at New York University Medical Center reported finding large-space-occupying abnormalities (such as tumors) in the cervical spine that produced no symptoms at all. As a result of these findings, they warned against attributing pain to bone spurs or herniated discs.

More recently, Joel Saal and several colleagues reported the successful nonsurgical treatment of twenty-four patients with herniated cervical discs and arm pain. None of the patients had worsening of their neurologic symptoms in the arm and most returned to normal physical activities. A similar study was reported by Keith Bush and his colleagues in London in 1996.

I have known of the innocence of the intervertebral disc for years but have not been able to report my findings except in my books. A paper documenting the cure of 88 percent of a group of TMS patients who had lumbar herniated disc has been rejected by seven medical journals.

Thoracic Outlet Syndrome

One of the diagnoses occasionally made when someone has pain of the shoulder and arm is thoracic outlet syndrome. The space traversed by the large blood vessel going into the arm is known as the thoracic outlet. The space can be narrowed by an extra rib, but this is quite rare. In the absence of an extra rib, doctors hypothesized that muscles in the shoulder are compressing the blood vessel and causing arm pain. There is no evidence that this happens. This is not to be confused with what happens in TMS, when reduced blood flow through thousands of tiny arterioles to an area that may include muscle and nerve results in mild oxygen deprivation. When this happens in the shoulder there is local muscle pain and there are nerve symptoms in the arm and hand because of involvement of nerves that go to the arm and hand. That is very different from what is being called thoracic outlet syndrome.

Repetitive Stress Injury

Like the low back pain problem, misdiagnosis and mismanagement have caused repetitive stress injury to assume epidemic proportions. In 1993 it was estimated that RSI was costing corporate America twenty billion dollars a year and was responsible for 56 percent of work-related illnesses. Carpal tunnel syndrome, one of the prominent components of RSI, was responsible for a 467 percent increase in disability claims in the United States between 1989 and 1994. Industry analysts are painfully aware that the problem has continued to increase since 1994.

As the term implies, symptoms are attributed to repetitive tasks, like working at a computer keyboard. In many cases muscle, nerve and tendon involvement are combined with symptoms in the neck, shoulders, arms and hands, often bilateral. Patients complain of pain, numbness, tingling and weakness, invariably brought on or aggravated by their job tasks. In many cases carpal tunnel syndrome is the primary diagnosis. Pain, numbness and tingling involve the hand and are attributed to compression of the median nerve by a band across the wrist, the flexor retinaculum. However, one expert on the subject has suggested that the manifestations of the disorders are better explained by the kind of minor vascular abnormality typical of TMS.

Here are some clinical histories of people with RSI:

➤ "Intense pain in both of my arms, sometimes feels better, but never goes away, so I can't do my regular job. It started two years ago at both elbows and gradually came to involve my hands, arms, shoulders and neck. I have trouble dressing and grooming myself. I have insomnia. I need lots of pillows to cushion my arms. Sex is very painful, so I don't have much interest. Household things are almost impossible, cooking, cleaning, shopping, laundry. It's hard for me to be much of a mother for my little boy. This thing invades every aspect of my life. Virtually everything I do with my arms or hands hurts. It's quite incredible."

➤ "I have been to ten doctors; most of them diagnosed carpal tunnel syndrome. I've been treated with physical therapy for a year, injections of cortisone that seemed to make it worse, and now they're talking about surgery."

➤ "In a few days it got so bad I couldn't lift my right arm. I thought I'd never type again. What was scary was the fact that no one seemed to get better from this. I'm somewhat better now, thanks to a great physical therapist, but I'm not cured. I have to be very careful how much I type. I spend a lot of time with my arms in ice."

➤ "I think this has been coming on for years. I remember having feelings of numbness in my

fingers at night and a strange sensation of weakness
in my arms. I'm better but I still have to be very
careful not to overdo."

Without the knowledge of TMS it would be impossible
to explain the symptoms. One patient said, "My neurologist
said it was a rheumatologic problem and my rheumatologist
said it was neurological."

One may well ask, What about the generations of women
(and some men) who worked at typewriters for years and
never developed RSI? They are like the millions of men and
women who did hard physical labor for years without having
severe problems with their backs or necks. People will develop mindbody manifestations that are in vogue. Fifty years
ago life's pressures might have produced stomach symptoms
or headaches. Today it is mostly back pain, RSI or chronic fatigue.

It is totally without logic to propose that after millions of
years of evolution, during which we have become the dominant species on this planet, our bodies have become structurally incompetent, or that we have become so fragile that
we must be careful how we move, use our bodies, or engage
in repetitive activities. This is unadulterated nonsense. We
are not made of papier-mâché; we are tough and resilient,
adaptable and quick to heal.

Another group of people who have suffered RSI symptoms for years, long before it was identified as a syndrome,
are musicians. How simple it is to blame the repetitive, intricate, often extremely fatiguing activities of a pianist or vio-
linist for neck, shoulder, arm and hand pain when one has
TMS.

I remember vividly a young concert cellist who came to
see me first for low back pain. When we succeeded in elimi-
nating that problem he began to have pain in various parts of

his arms, hands and shoulders, to the extent that his career was in jeopardy. Fortunately, he was very receptive to the idea of TMS, recovered completely, and has remained free of pain since 1988.

As with low back problems, an army of doctors and therapists confirms that symptoms of RSI are induced by purely physical factors and suggests many solutions based on avoiding supposedly injurious movements or postures. I wonder if the cellist would have come to me if his initial symptoms had been in the arms and hands instead of the back. Having had a successful experience with the back, he understood the brain's attempt to locate the pain in his arms and hands.

Conventional Treatment

Treatment for upper back, neck and arm syndromes is much the same as for low back pain, with a reliance on steroids or nonsteroidal anti-inflammatory medication, physical therapy, massage and other physical treatments. Many people have chiropractic manipulation, having been informed that they have a "subluxation," a minor dislocation. In my experience it is not possible to dislocate spinal elements except with violent trauma like a car accident. Any relief from such treatments must be based on the placebo phenomenon. Cervical collars are often prescribed as well as cervical traction. The former is supposed to immobilize the neck and the latter to pull the cervical vertebral bones apart. Surgery is commonly performed if there are neurological changes in an arm or hand with a herniated disc.

When TMS is the cause of symptoms, there is no rationale for any of the treatments, since they are predicated on a structural abnormality, or an inflammatory process that has never been identified. Complete and permanent elimination of pain depends on an accurate diagnosis.

5

Manifestations in Tendons

Knee Tendonitis

While virtually any tendon in the body may be the target for TMS, some are more frequently involved than others.

The knee is one of the most common sites. The pain may be anywhere in the front or back of the knee; a great many tendons attach around that joint. The largest is the patellar tendon, containing within it the patella (kneecap); it is the tendon of the quadriceps muscle, the weight-bearing muscle that keeps the knee from buckling during walking or running. The pain is usually in only part of the tendon, either above or below the kneecap. There are many others, including the hamstring tendons and those from muscles below the knee. The ligaments around the joint are important structures that help support it and may be a target for pain. All of this is easily ascertained on physical examination; the involved tendon hurts when you press on it. The problem does not involve the knee joint but the tendons attached to bones around the joint. Knee pain is often blamed on a condition known as chondromalacia. It is a roughening on the underside of the kneecap, diagnosed by X ray and, in my experience, painless. Once more we have a situation in which an X-ray abnormality is blamed for pain because the doctor is unaware of the existence of TMS. Pain may also be attributed to an unstable patella, or that old standby, arthritis. Occasionally a small tear in a meniscus (cartilage) is said to be the cause of the pain. Meniscus tears can be seen on imaging studies and are very often painless but will be blamed for pain really caused by TMS tendonitis. Not uncommonly these patients have arthroscopic surgery. I saw such a patient recently. After the arthroscopic procedure he continued to have pain, so the surgeon did a second one on the grounds that a fold of tissue was causing the pain. But the pain continued. Though this patient came to see me for his back, I informed him of the true nature of his knee pain and he was able to solve both problems simultaneously.

Although it is less common, swelling of the knee may accompany tendonitis. When I first became aware of this I felt a little insecure about advising the patient that it was part of TMS. In the light of consistent success in treatment, I am now quite comfortable with that diagnosis.

Shoulder Tendonitis

The shoulder is a frequent TMS site. Diagnosis can be complicated, as pain in this area may be due to brachial plexus involvement, described in Chapter 4. It is often part of RSI.

The diagnostic history of pain in this region (where the arm meets the shoulder) is interesting. Before the advent of magnetic resonance imaging (MRI), the procedure that allows precise diagnosis of a rotator cuff tear, the most common diagnoses were bursitis and calcium deposits. The latter diagnosis often led to surgical removal. Now the diagnosis made most frequently is rotator cuff tear.

I never thought to challenge that condition as a cause of pain until the following experience with a patient. She was a woman in her fifties who had been treated successfully for back pain years earlier. She called to tell me she had developed pain in one of her shoulders and had consulted a number of the best orthopedists in town. Because an MRI showed a rotator cuff tear, she had surgery. Now, although the pain was relieved, she was beginning to experience the same pain in the opposite shoulder and wondered if this could be a manifestation of TMS. I said I thought it likely and arranged an appointment for an examination. She came in a few days later and reported that the pain had disappeared overnight after we had talked. There was still mild tenderness when I pressed on one of the tendons at the shoulder.

This was an important experience for me. To be sure, torn tendons require repair, especially in athletes like baseball pitchers, but here again is a situation where doctors treat X rays rather than patients. It is my practice now to treat shoulder pain as TMS if a painful tendon is found on examination. Moreover, the medical literature suggests that rotator cuff tears may be part of the aging process, like the arthritic changes in the spine that are always mistakenly blamed for pain.

I have often said that the MRI has been a mixed blessing for people with pain syndromes. The herniated disc, the torn meniscus in the knee and the rotator cuff tear at the shoulders, all dependent on MRI for identification, have resulted in much well-meaning but needless surgery.

Tennis Elbow

Here is an old favorite that has been eclipsed in recent years by the more dramatic knee problems and rotator cuff tears. Bear in mind that TMS requires only one pain location at a time. If knee or shoulder pain occur more frequently, the incidence of elbow pain may diminish. However, it is still common and may, like other locations in the arm, be part of RSI. As most people now know, tennis elbow occurs in many people who do not play tennis. It is still regarded as a strain on a tendon attaching a muscle to a bone at the elbow. Rest and immobilization are the usual treatments; steroid injections are often employed. Like all TMS manifestations, tennis elbow responds well to the program of education once the patient has accepted the fact that the pain is due to TMS.

Tendonitis of the Foot

The foot is a very important TMS location. Anyone who has suffered foot pain knows it can be quite disabling. There are many tendons on top of the foot and around the ankle, any of which can be the target for TMS. Pain occurs more frequently on the bottom than on the top of the foot. Toward the front it is called metatarsalgia and is often attributed to a neuroma (a benign nerve tumor); surgical excision of the neuroma is not uncommon. When the pain is in the arch it is called plantar fasciitis; in the heel it is often attributed to a bone spur if one is found on X ray. Because patients have a harder time accepting that foot pain is part of TMS, it tends to linger.

Flat feet are often mistakenly blamed for foot pain.

Shin Splints

A familiar term to athletes, trainers and doctors in sports medicine, *shin splints* refers to pain along the front of the leg, between the knee and the foot. Like so many common pain syndromes, it has been a diagnostic mystery. Usually associated with athletic activity, it is another example of TMS tendonitis. Recent studies have shown X-ray changes in the tibial bone but I am still inclined to attribute the pain to TMS.

The tibia, the major leg bone below the knee, is easily felt in front of the lower leg, for it lies just under the skin. Attached to it along much of its length is the important tibialis anterior muscle. It can be felt in the right leg just to the right of the tibia. This muscle has primary responsibility for elevating the front of the foot during the gait or run cycle: Its importance is obvious. (To feel soreness in this muscle, walk as fast as you can for at least thirty minutes.) People with shin splints experience pain if you press on this muscle. The tendon of the tibialis anterior muscle is attached to the tibial bone along its entire length. Shin splints are TMS tendonitis. Soreness from muscular activity will pass in a day or two. When the pain persists and intensifies, it means that superimposed TMS is the cause.

Pulled Hamstring

A common occurrence among even superbly conditioned athletes is sudden pain in the back of the thigh while actively engaged in a sport. Because of the acute onset, muscle injury is assumed to be the culprit.

Having noted a number of pulled hamstrings in professional football games, and considering the circumstances in which they occurred and the relatively rapid recovery of the athletes, I am strongly inclined to the idea that the players are experiencing acute attacks of TMS tendonitis. I particularly recall one football player who sustained a pulled hamstring in a game. He was said to have been treated vigorously in preparation for the next game, and indeed he was able to start the following week. He played most of that game but sometime late in the third quarter had to come out again for a pulled hamstring—this time in the other leg. When asked by reporters what he thought had happened, he said he had overused that leg because of having injured the other one the week before. That is a ridiculous idea; there was no change in his run, no evidence of a limp. I watched him carefully and could see no reason for an injury when he developed the new pain—he simply "pulled up lame." This was a very high-strung man, the star of his team, upon whom everyone counted. The pressure on him must have been enormous. Little wonder that he was prone to frequent episodes of TMS.

Coccydynia (Coccygodynia, Coccyalgia)

A number of less common tendonitises are also manifestations of TMS. In coccydynia, the tendons involved are of muscles that attach to various pelvic bones and to the sacrum and coccyx. The sacrum and coccyx are often thought of as extensions of the lumbar spine. The coccyx is all that is left of the tail in humans and other advanced mammals like chimpanzees. The pain is experienced in the cleft between the gluteal muscles and is most likely due to TMS involvement of the tendons of muscles attaching to the sacrum, rather than the coccyx. It behaves as low back symptoms do: The pain may occur under peculiar circumstances, although, as expected, sitting invariably brings it on.

Less commonly, the tendons of muscles in the thigh that attach to pelvic bones, like the hamstrings and adductors of the thigh, are involved. In most cases the tendons are painful to finger pressure. I have had patients with involvement of the tough ligament in the groin, the inguinal ligament. Any tendon or ligament in the body can be the target for TMS.

This concludes the description of the muscle, nerve and tendon manifestations of TMS. Let us look now at one of the most distressing consequences of these pain syndromes, chronic pain, and one of the most bizarre, Lyme disease.

6

Chronic Pain and Lyme Disease

Chronic Pain

I can still recall our attempts at the then Institute of Rehabilitation Medicine, New York University Medical Center, to establish a program for the treatment of chronic pain many years ago. Since I was beginning to realize that most back pain was psychologically induced and the medical literature was suggesting that chronic pain was the result of psychological factors, establishing a program to treat chronic pain seemed like a good thing to pursue. Accordingly, we followed the guidelines recommended by the experts, set up a multidisciplinary team consisting of physical therapist, occupational therapist, nurse, psychologist, social worker and doctor, and proceeded to admit patients to the program. The patients we treated suffered from various painful structural conditions, including arthritis of the spine, a herniated disc, and fibrositis (now called fibromyalgia). Their pain had continued for more than six months despite treatment and was so severe it dominated their lives. It prevented work and normal social intercourse and led to a host of personal problems. In most cases the patients were taking a variety of drugs in high dosages.

The postulated psychological factor central to the therapeutic program was that patients were deriving *secondary gain* from the pain, meaning that unconsciously they needed the pain to continue so they could be cared for, avoid responsibility or work or perhaps get money. Most patients were anxious and depressed, had trouble sleeping, ate poorly and looked ill. They were clearly not malingering; the secondary gain was said to be unconscious. Chronic pain was proclaimed to be a disease entity unto itself.

Based on these observations the program developed as follows:

1. Psychological testing on admission
2. Evaluation by each member of the team to determine what his or her contribution to the recovery process would be
3. No discussion of pain or reward for pain behavior
4. Stimulation of physical, vocational and social activities
5. Identification and treatment of psychological and social problems
6. Creation of a "cocktail" of drugs the patient had been taking, and the gradual reduction of the component amounts without the patient's knowledge

We all participated in the program with great enthusiasm. It was perfect for rehabilitation medicine because we routinely worked as a team to treat many disabling conditions. Before long we began to suspect that the postulated psychological basis for the condition was flawed. Our psychological evaluations suggested that there were, indeed, powerful psychological factors at work to perpetuate the pain, but they did not precipitate secondary gain. A good example was a woman who had suffered childhood sexual and emotional abuse so severe that we marveled she had survived it. She was almost totally disabled by pain, so great was the rage she carried in her unconscious.

Increasingly, we discussed the pain with the patient, where it came from and why it would go away once the psychological poison was revealed. We found it wasn't necessary to surreptitiously reduce drugs; the patients stopped taking them spontaneously. And, of course, the physiologic explanation for the pain had emerged. Chronic pain was TMS in one of its most severe forms. There was no need to formulate a separate disease entity called chronic pain.

That was about twenty years ago and time has only reinforced our conclusions.

What is the status of diagnosis and treatment of continuing, severe pain today? There are pain centers all over the country carrying on programs for chronic pain based on the idea of secondary gain. These programs have the approval of doctors and official psychiatric and psychological associations. The *Diagnostic and Statistical Manual for Mental Disorders* specifies pain disorder as one of a number of somatoform disorders but does not identify unconscious factors as the cause of pain. The word *somatoform* identifies the malady as physical.

Some practitioners, however, are giving emotions more credence. In an article in the *New York Times*, December 12, 1992, "Chronic Pain Fells Many Yet Lacks Clear Cause," Elisabeth Rosenthal quoted a well-known student of the problems of pain, Dr. John Loeser of the University of Washington: "All the evidence suggests that for most people chronic pain is a stress-related disorder, just like ulcers. The difference with pain is that we don't know where to put the tube to look."

In the same article another expert was quoted: "Maybe it's not really pain but a metaphor for anxiety or depression or spiritual suffering. We use 'pain' for physical and emotional distress, and sometimes people don't make the distinction very well."

Here is clear evidence that thoughtful people in medicine recognize the psychological basis for chronic pain. Nevertheless, this is only the beginning. Medicine has yet to acknowledge the process whereby strong unconscious emotions induce physical reactions. Without that knowledge the profession is diagnostically at sea and the epidemic continues.

Lyme Disease

Although it differs considerably from those already discussed, another medical condition warrants mention. In this case we have a bona fide disease process to which a variety of physical symptoms are mistakenly attributed. Lyme disease is a bacterial infection acquired through the bite of a tiny tick that can manifest itself in neurological and arthritic symptoms. If someone has pain that cannot be explained by any of the usual diagnoses and has immunologic evidence (from a blood test) of having been infected, the symptoms will be attributed to Lyme disease. Whenever a foreign substance like a bacterium enters the body, the immune system activates protective measures. One of these is the creation of substances called antibodies that link up with the bacteria and neutralize them. Antibodies are specific for each bacterium; each of us has many different antibodies circulating in our blood. The amount of a specific antibody can be measured in the laboratory. The amount is known as an antibody titer. By this test one can determine whether or not an antibody for a specific disease is present in the blood, and how much. I have seen many people with TMS whose pain was attributed to Lyme disease because they had antibodies for the Lyme bacterium in their blood.

One of many cases I encountered was a man I saw with severe TMS who did not accept that diagnosis and was later found to have antibodies for Lyme disease. He sued the neurologists who had attended him originally for malpractice, claiming that they had failed to test for Lyme antibodies. His symptoms were blatantly TMS, but in the absence of medical acceptance of TMS the neurologists found it difficult to defend themselves.

7

The Equivalents of TMS

Physical reactions to emotional states are the stuff of everyday life. You have a close call on the highway and your heart begins to pound. You are getting up to address an audience and your mouth is dry; you have butterflies in the stomach. The perspiration flows freely in a tight situation. You repress a sudden rage and all of these reactions happen at once.

The body is intimately connected to the mind, and particularly to emotions. How could it be otherwise?

The disorders I will describe now are a bit more complicated than the ones I have mentioned thus far, and all appear to serve the same purpose as TMS. That is, they are designed to be distractions from unconscious rage.

Many physical conditions are TMS equivalents. Like the pain syndromes, the majority of these are basically harmless. They fall into seven categories, disorders of:

1. The gastrointestinal system
2. The circulatory system
3. The skin
4. The immune system
5. The genitourinary system
6. The cardiac mechanism
7. Miscellaneous

With all of these disorders it is essential to consult your regular physician and rule out serious disease.

Gastrointestinal Disorders

For many years gastrointestinal (GI) disorders were the most common of the emotionally induced physical conditions.

Upper GI Disturbances

The esophagus at the top of the GI tract may be the site of spasm, perceived as an aching pain in the chest right under the breastbone. It feels as though the lower end of the esophagus is being squeezed. In a more serious disorder, there is constriction at the esophageal junction with the stomach, sometimes requiring surgical release. Food is not passed into the stomach and is regurgitated. This condition is not common.

Stomach symptoms, however, are common. One of the most prevalent, heartburn, is caused by hyperacidity and can be alleviated with antacid preparations. Rumination, the regurgitation of small amounts of food after a meal, is fairly common. Mild stomach discomfort is often attributed to gastritis. Some of these symptoms have been associated with what is known as hiatus hernia. Heartburn and upper abdominal discomfort when recumbent are said to be the result of herniation of a small part of the upper stomach into the chest cavity when lying flat. It can be identified on X ray. Conventional treatment consists of taking antacids and elevating the head of the bed.

It is my belief that all upper GI symptoms can be equivalents of TMS, therefore psychologically induced. Because hiatus hernia is a structural abnormality, one can understand reluctance to attribute it to emotional factors. However, no one has ever explained the process that produces a hiatus hernia. Its association with heartburn and esophageal reflux suggests that it, too, is an equivalent of TMS.

Though not as common as they used to be, peptic ulcers of the stomach or duodenum are still a medical problem. The discovery that people with ulcers often (but not always) harbor a bacterium, *Helicobacter pylori,* in their stomachs has aroused great interest. The bacterium is currently regarded as the cause of stomach and duodenal ulcers. But then how does one explain the ulcer when the bacterium is not found in the stomach of someone with an ulcer? The *New York Times* recently reported (August 7, 1997) that scientists have suggested that the bacterium *Helicobacter pylori* has been a benign inhabitant of the intestinal tracts of human beings and our evolutionary predecessors for millions of years. Why should this harmless bacteria suddenly become pathological? In my view it is not. Its presence in the stomach of some people with ulcers does not mean that it is the cause of those ulcers. It may simply be part of the still somewhat mysterious process whereby an ulcer develops. What is clear to me is that emotional factors initiate that process.

The willingness of contemporary medicine to accept the bacterial explanation of the cause of ulcers is another example of its philosophical bias that emotions do not initiate physical disorders.

Serious disorders like cancer should always be ruled out before one concludes that stomach symptoms are stress-induced. This is true of every painful condition. Fortunately, benign stomach ulcers are far more common than malignant ones.

The following incident is an excellent illustration of the emotionally induced nature of stomach disorders. A gentleman in his mid-forties accompanied his wife, who was my patient, to a teaching session during which I talked about the many equivalents of TMS. A few weeks later I received a letter from the man telling me that the stomach symptoms he had suffered every day of his life for the past twenty-five years were gone. He understood and accepted the principle of psychological causation as applicable to his symptoms—and he got better.

Another source of stomach pain is spasm of the pylorus, the muscular tissue at the outlet of the stomach which acts as a sphincter, preventing or allowing the passage of food from the stomach into the small intestine. This, too, is a TMS equivalent.

Lower GI Disorders

Diarrhea or frequent bowel movements have long been associated with "being nervous" or having a "nervous stomach." Bowel irregularities, abdominal pain, cramps and excessive gas give rise to the diagnoses spastic colon, colitis and irritable bowel syndrome. All of these, as well as constipation, are largely psychological in origin.

Like TMS, gastrointestinal maladies are brought about by the autonomic nervous system. Many symptoms are the result of alterations in the normal motility of the lower tract, producing frequent, loose bowel movements when motility is increased and constipation when it is decreased. *Motility* refers to the peristaltic action (muscular contractions) in the intestine that moves solid materials along. If peristalsis stops completely, or the bowel spasms, painful symptoms occur.

All of these changes are the result of the psychological process described in Chapter 1.

Disorders of the Circulatory System

Tension Headache, Migraine Headache, Raynaud's Phenomenon

Tension and migraine headache are very common and sometimes confused, since unilateral, severe headache, often accompanied by nausea and vomiting, is characteristic of migraine but often occurs with severe tension headache. Although they may seem similar, migraine patients frequently experience a visual phenomenon just before the headache begins. Technically called scintillating scotoma, it is a disturbing, usually shimmering, jagged line in the peripheral visual field that lasts for about fifteen minutes.

Tension headache is classed as a circulatory disorder, since it is believed that the headache is caused by local ischemia in the scalp muscles, just as TMS comes from local ischemia in postural muscles, nerves or tendons.

Migraine, on the other hand, is thought to be caused by sudden constriction of a single blood vessel within the substance of the brain. That sounds ominous but it rarely leads to anything more serious than a headache.

My own experience with migraine many years ago made its relation to psychological factors very plain. As a young doctor in family practice with the usual stresses and strains of work and family, I suffered from migraines for about six years. A colleague told me of a medical paper he had read suggesting that migraine headache was the result of repressed anger. Since I was coming to the conclusion that psychological factors were very common in day-to-day medical problems, I was receptive to that idea. When next the premonitory "lights" began, I sat down and thought about what anger I might be repressing. Years later it is clear to me what I was repressing, but at the time I had no idea. However, to my astonishment, the headache never came. Nor have I ever had another migraine headache, though I have continued to have the "dancing lights" to this day. The "lights" tell me that I am repressing anger, and sometimes I have to think very hard to figure out the reason for the anger. Often it is obvious.

A very important lesson is to be learned from this experience, one that applies to TMS and all its equivalents: In many cases merely acknowledging that a symptom may be emotional in origin is enough to stop it. I didn't know what I was unconsciously angry about, but I was willing to accept that something psychological was responsible for my headache. That alone prevented the migraine permanently.

I encountered the same thing when I began to make the TMS diagnosis, though I did not relate it to my migraine experience at the time. I would tell patients their backaches were induced by stress and tension, and if they were open to that idea, they got better. For many years, although I understood this approach worked, I didn't understand why. The explanation is in Parts I and III of this book. But the significance of the observation should not be lost: A physical symptom is eliminated by the process of thought. It is not a magical phenomenon. By shifting one's attention from the realm of the physical to that of the psychological, a physical symptom is banished. I personally have done it with migraine headache, pollen allergies, gastrointestinal symptoms and skin reactions. My patients frequently report similar experiences, as do their spouses.

The last of the circulatory disorders, Raynaud's phenomenon, refers to the tendency for people's extremities, hands and feet to react excessively to cold and become whitish or even blue. This is a psychologically induced overreaction to the autonomic system's normal response to cold by restricting circulation of blood to the extremities in order to conserve heat. This is yet another example of hyperactivity of the autonomic nervous system in response to emotional stimuli.

Skin Disorders

I suspect that many skin conditions—commonly acne, eczema, hives and psoriasis—are emotionally induced, an idea that most practicing dermatologists would reject.

Work being done in the laboratories of research dermatologists would tend to support that assertion. Research workers in the Department of Dermatology of the University of Pennsylvania School of Medicine found evidence of a potential link between brain factors and a cellular inflammatory response seen commonly in a variety of skin disorders. According to a report published by members of the department, "Such a link could have clinical significance in the commonly observed exacerbation of many dermatoses, such as psoriasis and atopic disease, by emotional stress." Although direct proof of the connection between emotional states and specific dermatologic disorders has not been found, such studies provide compelling evidence that the discovery will be made.

My clinical experience shows that the emotional stress in these physical disorders is not necessarily a result of external causes. It is an internal process resulting in strong feelings that the unconscious mind considers to be dangerous and threatening and which, therefore, must be repressed. As described in Part I of this book, physical symptoms play a role in the process of repression.

The dermatologic study just noted is extremely important because it begins to bridge the gap that proclaims that the mind and the body are separate entities having nothing to do with each other.

Disorders of the Immune System

Medical scientists are slowly coming to the conclusion that important connections exist between emotional processes and a variety of physical systems, such as the endocrine network and the immune system. Some of the most exciting work is being done by those interested in the immune system. An article in the *New England Journal of Medicine* found that "central nervous system influences on the immune system are well documented and provide a mechanism by which emotional states could influence the course of diseases involving immune function. Whether emotional factors can influence the course of autoimmune disease, cancer, and infection in humans is a subject of intense research that has not been satisfactorily resolved at this time."

I will discuss autoimmune disorders and cancer later. For the moment let's look at a group of benign maladies that are examples of how emotions affect immune functions.

Allergies

In allergic reactions to pollens, dust and molds, the immune system overreacts to the foreign substance, producing the well-known symptoms of itchy eyes, sneezing and nasal discharge and clogging. Asthma may have a similar cause, although the emotions may exert a direct effect on the respiratory mechanism by constricting the bronchioles, creating wheezing and difficulty in breathing.

Allergic reactions in infants are the result of a different process whose cause is unknown.

Another example of hypersensitivity is hives (urticaria or angioedema). Most often it consists of itchy bumps, but it may be more extensive, with swelling of large segments of skin and underlying tissue. Sometimes hives are part of an explosive reaction called anaphylaxis, which induces respiratory distress and vascular collapse. Hives alone or anaphylaxis are thought to be reactions to ingested food or substances injected by human or insect. Medical textbooks tell us that these reactions are allergic but do not state what initiates the process.

People may have adverse reactions to foreign substances injected into the body. An October 1974 issue of *Medical*

World News reported that a Cleveland radiologist had concluded that allergic reactions (nausea, vomiting, hives and sometimes life-threatening anaphylaxis) to dye injected for X-ray studies of the renal system were not allergic at all but were emotional, caused by "ubiquitous and unreasonable" fear. Dr. Lalli found that when he allayed his patients' fear with a "calm, self-assured approach, augmented by an easy manner and casual conversation," he was able to perform repeated urographic examinations, even on patients with a history of severe reactions, with no difficulty. Dr. Lalli documented his experience in a paper published in the journal *Radiology*.

My personal experience with hives is instructive. After joining the Army in 1943, I volunteered for the Air Corps. While I was doing coursework at the University of Alabama and ten hours of flight instruction in a light plane, I began to awaken in the morning with giant hives on my face. On testing, the Army doctor found me allergic to a large number of foods, all of which I then studiously avoided, but I continued to have the hives. We moved to a station in Texas for classification (as pilot, navigator or bombardier), where we were informed that the Air Corps had decided it had all the people it needed. We were all sent back from whence we came—in my case to the Medical Department. The attacks of hives stopped.

My experience is a prime example of the two minds we have talked about. My conscious mind wanted to fight the Nazis. The response of my unconscious mind was, "Don't you realize that flying in combat is dangerous? Are you crazy?" That induced the sequence of physiological events that culminated in hives.

Did the foods to which I tested allergic play a role? The same question may be asked of someone who has a severe reaction to an insect bite. Obviously there is a connection, but the sting or the food are clearly not causative; they are part of the process. An unconscious emotion causes the immune system to react to the food or wasp sting.

Medical science continues to learn about the details of allergic reactions and about how the immune system functions. It is a very complicated system; we must be careful not to confuse the intricate parts and functions of a machine with what makes it go in the first place. Electricity makes an electric motor run, not its parts.

Modern medical science studies the details of maladies but rejects unconscious emotional processes as the cause. When mainstream medicine does study a possible psychological role in causation, it tends to look at perceived emotions like anxiety and depression and relies on psychological profiles to categorize people. Unfortunately, perceived emotions and profiles may tell us nothing about what is going on in the unconscious.

If someone had given me a personality inventory when I was having the hives, they would have learned nothing. I was a young man, gung-ho to fight the enemy; I truly enjoyed flying and I was neither anxious nor depressed. On the other hand, an analytically oriented psychiatrist or psychologist who suspected the emotional source of the hives would soon have discovered what was going on in my mind. Not everyone, however, needs a psychotherapist to find out what's going on when they have TMS or one of its equivalents— most people need simple knowledge. Everyone generates unconscious feelings; sometimes they are troubling enough to stimulate physical symptoms.

Infections

The second group of emotionally induced immune system reactions reflects an inadequate or idiosyncratic response to infectious agents. Frequent colds or urinary tract infections, recurrent herpes simplex, yeast infections, prostatitis, acne—all are examples of an inadequate immune response to an invader.

Infections are perhaps even more common than allergic reactions but are rarely recognized as psychogenic because we have become so accustomed to thinking of a malady only in terms of the infectious agent that produces it. Colds are caused by viruses, as are influenza and a host of other maladies. A sore throat is caused by a virus, with or without a bacterium like the streptococcus; meningitis is caused by a variety of organisms, pneumonia by others. We take steps to avoid contact with germs; we receive inoculations to protect us from them and we search for antibiotics to kill them. All are medically sound ideas.

For all our efforts to avoid illness, however, nothing is done to improve function in the immune system, the system that ultimately overcomes the infection, with or without antibiotics, or prevents it in the first place. This is the Department of Defense for your body. Its weapons include chemicals, clever contraptions that link up with the infectious agent and nullify it, and cells that destroy the invader or swallow it up. The immune system is quite amazing, but then it has been about 570 million years in the making, so I suppose we shouldn't be surprised at its efficiency.

My clinical experience indicates that emotions can enhance, modify or reduce the efficiency of immune system function. The science of these processes has yet to be explained; they are waiting to be studied.

The Epstein-Barr Syndrome

Epstein-Barr syndrome is an ill-defined disorder characterized by fatigue and a variety of aches and pains. It derives its name from the fact that some people with these symptoms have been found to have an elevated antibody titer for the Epstein-Barr virus. (The Epstein-Barr virus is the one that causes infectious mononucleosis, so it is likely that we all have antibodies against this virus in our bloodstreams.) Many of my patients with TMS reported having had such elevated titers and were told they suffered from the Epstein-Barr syndrome.

Growing evidence suggests that Epstein-Barr antibody titers are affected by psychological processes. A paper published in the *Journal of Consulting and Clinical Psychology* in 1994 reported a *decrease in antibody titers for the Epstein-Barr virus* in people who were given the opportunity to write or speak about feelings that had been hitherto repressed. In another study, people who wrote about their feelings about a stressful event produced increased numbers of lymphocytes, one of the immune system's cells that combat infection. These studies clearly point to the role of emotions in modifying immune system function.

This finding is of great public health importance. Disability claims based on the Epstein-Barr syndrome increased 320 percent between 1989 and 1994. The syndrome appears to be a combination of immune system malfunction (giving rise to the elevated antibody titers) and TMS symptoms, both of which can be attributed to the emotional process described in Part I of this book.

Genitourinary Disorders

Perhaps the most common genitourinary disorder is frequent urination, particularly at night. According to conventional medical wisdom, nocturia may be a significant symptom indicative of diabetes, cardiac disease, kidney disease or other more exotic disorders, so it should be taken seriously and studied by your physician. In most cases nothing will be found. In that case you may assume that the symptom is psychologically induced, especially if you have a history of other psychogenic processes, like TMS or GI disturbances.

Frequent infections of the lower urinary tract were mentioned in the section on the immune system. They should be treated with antibiotics if necessary, but good management includes attention to psychological factors, since they are basically responsible for the infection, having reduced the efficiency of the immune system and allowed the infectious agent to take hold.

Prostatitis is frequently induced by stress factors. It includes symptoms like discomfort, mild pain and burning upon urination. There is often no evidence of infection. Urologists also know that loss of libido and various forms of impotence may be the result of psychological factors. It should, therefore, not be surprising that studies often fail to disclose a physical reason for the impotence.

Disorders of the Cardiac Mechanism

The equivalents of TMS in this category have to do with aberrations in heart rate and rhythm.

Paroxysmal auricular tachycardia is characterized by a very rapid heart rate that starts suddenly and, in my experience, is precipitated by an emotional situation. Medical intervention is required to bring the heart rate back to normal if that doesn't happen spontaneously.

Ectopic, or extra, beats are very common and appear to be the result of more subtle unconscious emotions, judging by my personal experience with the disorder. They should always be evaluated to rule out cardiac disease. Though more common at rest, they can occur in the course of vigorous physical activity. Ectopic beats in someone with mitral valve prolapse are erroneously attributed to the prolapse. They are related only in that both are the consequence of stress factors. There will be more about mitral valve prolapse in the appropriate section later in this book.

Miscellaneous Disorders

Hypoglycemia

Hypoglycemia (low blood sugar) is another condition whose psychogenic origin is hard to prove. I can only set forth the idea, based on anecdotal evidence, that hypoglycemia is emotionally induced. I experience it from time to time but it never persists because I am aware of its cause. Like all psychogenic symptoms, it is very susceptible to placebo suggestion; thus altering the diet, although it does not cure hypoglycemia, often causes it to abate.

Dizziness

Although dizziness is frequently attributed to an infection in the semicircular canals, in my experience most cases of dizziness, including people with true vertigo, are stress-induced. Naturally, dizziness should be studied by appropriate specialists, but when no other cause is found (as is usually the case), the true cause is obvious. Unfortunately, failure to recognize the psychogenic nature of the problem often leads to treatments that help to perpetuate rather than alleviate symptoms. The treatments may be benign but foster the idea that an infectious agent is responsible, thus allowing the mind to continue the distraction. I have had patients whose dizziness disappeared promptly when they learned that it was psychologically induced.

Tinnitus

This is a very disturbing symptom, commonly referred to as "ringing in the ears." It can be a sign of an ear or neurologic disorder and should always be thoroughly investigated by the appropriate specialists. If no other cause is found, one may safely assume that it is a TMS equivalent. Many patients with TMS have reported having had the symptom at some time in the past and noted that it disappeared when their back pain began. It is hard to avoid the conclusion that it is serving the same psychologic purpose as TMS.

Chronic Fatigue Syndrome

This disorder continues to mystify a medical community that can neither define it nor identify its cause. Fatigue, nonspecific aches and pains, chronic infection and failure to find laboratory or physical signs pathognomonic of the disorder leave medicine frustrated and impotent. Difficulty concentrating, mood disturbances and depression have been noted in many patients with CFS but, students of the problem complain, no diagnoses in the *Diagnostic and Statistical Manual of Mental Disorders* identify the person with CFS, implying that it is not a mental disorder.

Both the nonpsychiatric and psychiatric communities reject the concept of psychogenicity; as I have said before, the word *psychosomatic* does not appear in *DSM-IV*. Except for conversion symptoms, now rare, medicine does not believe that unconscious phenomena induce physical symptoms. Practitioners are doomed, therefore, to remain ignorant of the cause of such maladies as CFS and the Epstein-Barr syndrome. Research on CFS, fibromyalgia and myofascial pain identifies similarities in these disorders for good reason— their cause is the same.

A comprehensive review of all aspects of CFS was published as the report of a joint working group of three Royal Colleges—Physicians, Psychiatrists and General Practitioners—in October 1996. Drawing from published research as well as their own clinical experience, they explored the definition of CFS, possible causes, diagnostic tests to perform on patients with the syndrome and treatment.

The group was unable to identify a disease process (e.g., infection, cancer, etc.) as possible cause, but found that over half of people with CFS had one or more of the following: depression, sleep disturbance, poor concentration, agitation, feelings of worthlessness, guilt, suicidal thoughts and appetite or weight change. An additional 25 percent suffered from anxiety and what the investigating panel call somatization disorders, physical symptoms that are associated with depression and anxiety.

The report emphasized that practitioners must accept the symptoms as real (as opposed to imaginary or hypochondriacal). The most promising therapeutic approaches were gradually increased physical activity and cognitive behavior therapy, a form of psychotherapy that aims to "increase activity, reduce avoidance behavior, improve confidence and illness control, reevaluate the understanding of illness, combat depression and anxiety and look for underlying patterns of thoughts and assumptions that may contribute to disability."

Though not quite on target, this report is an important document. It points in the direction of psychology as the dominant factor in CFS, both in its cause and treatment. Practitioners should recognize that both psychological and physical symptoms may be the result of strong unconscious feelings. Pain, fatigue, anxiety and depression are all symptoms. The therapeutic approach should be cognitive-analytic. You cannot "combat" anxiety and depression; you must find

the reasons for them. When patients confront the unconscious feelings responsible for their symptoms, the symptoms
disappear.

Spasmodic Dysphonia

Spasmodic dysphonia, formerly called spastic dysphonia, is a
voice disorder that is caused by spasm of the vocal cords
(laryngospasm). For many years it was thought to be psychological in origin but, as with so many other maladies, contemporary students of the problem think that most cases are
neurogenic, that is, the result of a brain disorder. Some cases
are still diagnosed as psychogenic, however, and in other
cases the cause is not clear (idiopathic).

There are two main types of spasmodic dysphonia (SD):
the adductor form, in which the vocal cords stay more or less
closed, producing a strained, squeezed, jerky kind of speech;
and the abductor form, where the cords are kept apart so that
the voice sounds breathy, or disappears intermittently.

Based on the few patients I have seen who have suffered
from SD, all of whom had back pain syndromes, my suspi-
cion is that most cases of spasmodic dysphonia are psychogenic but are not identified as such because the person is
not suffering any obvious psychological problem. The significant emotions are repressed in the unconscious.

The difficulty with research on conditions like TMS and
SD is that psychometric tests do not reveal the presence of repressed feelings. Understandably, those feelings that are most
painful and undesirable will be most deeply repressed and
hardest to get at.

An excellent study published in the *Journal of Communication Disorders* illustrates the research problem. The author
found that ten of eighteen patients with SD were either anx-

ious or depressed and five of the ten were both. In addition, SD patients complained of physical symptoms more than their counterparts in a control group, who were matched for age, sex and whether they were right- or left-handed.

From my vantage point, the study did not disclose the psychological reason for the SD in any of the patients because it did not reveal what was being repressed in the unconscious. The anxiety or depression found in the ten was obviously a reflection of a more basic problem in the unconscious that produced the anxiety or depression.

Analytically oriented psychologists and psychiatrists are criticized for not producing objective data to support their conclusions about psychosomatic disorders. Unfortunately, most psychometric measures are useless because what they measure is not relevant to the problem at hand. Bringing powerful, frightening feelings to light can only be done by a skilled therapist. I cannot imagine a psychometric test that could do the same thing, though I'm sure it would be a boon to humanity if someone could design it.

In addition to those discussed here, a large number of psychologically induced physical disorders are less common but equally disabling. Undiagnosed ophthalmic conditions, the dry mouth syndrome and idiopathic laryngitis, for example, are psychogenic. I believe no organ or system in the body is immune from psychogenic involvement.

It is important to avoid the pejorative conclusion that because emotions are implicated in etiology, patients are making themselves sick. This is no more logical than feeling guilty for "letting" bacteria into the body. People with psychogenic illness are not deliberately making themselves sick or pretending to be unwell. What we are seeing is the interplay of complicated processes, both physiological and psychological, outside of conscious awareness and control. Many genetic and environmental factors contribute to the finished product called personality. Its development is an exceedingly complex process that we are only beginning to understand. To feel guilty over emotionally induced disorders is both pointless and illogical. Happily, learning about one's emotions and how they lead to body dysfunction is actually therapeutic. That is the lesson I have learned in my experience with TMS and its equivalents.

The disorders just described under the headings of TMS and its equivalents are without doubt responsible for a substantial proportion of the Western world's medical ills. Their proper management would alleviate much suffering and reduce the enormous cost of medical care that now burdens modern society.

8

Disorders in which Emotions
May Play a Role

While there is a clear and direct relation between emotions and TMS and its equivalents, there are only suggestive observations that unconscious processes participate in the genesis of the disorders we are about to discuss. Because they are more serious and often life threatening, the possibility that emotions may play an important etiologic role mandates intensive study. I believe much of the research that has been done on these conditions is flawed because it does not consider the possibility that emotions may contribute to their onset and, therefore, does not include that factor in research design. Recent research has left little doubt that the brain is intimately involved in a variety of body systems previously thought to function autonomously. However, researchers consider emotional factors only in the context of their influence on the *course* of autoimmune disease, cancer or infection—not their *cause*.

Autoimmune Disorders

In contrast to TMS and its equivalents, autoimmune disorders are characterized by pathological alteration of tissue that is more or less permanent. This is particularly diabolical because the tissue-destructive processes are generated in the person's own body, hence the designation *auto*. Autoimmune diseases appear to be examples of malevolent malfunction in the immune system.

The group includes rheumatoid arthritis, multiple sclerosis, diabetes, Grave's disease, periarteritis nodosa, lupus erythematosis, myasthenia gravis, hemolytic anemia, thrombocytopenic purpura, pernicious anemia, idiopathic Addison's disease, glomerulonephritis, Sjogren's syndrome, Guillain-Barré syndrome, some cases of infertility and possibly a large number of other disorders. It is beyond the scope of this book to describe these diseases.

Considerable research demonstrates the variety of ways in which the brain can modulate the immune system. For example, the multiple hormones secreted by the pituitary gland that have direct and indirect effects on the immune system are under the control of the hypothalamus, which in turn can be influenced by higher brain levels (suprahypothalamic), those having to do with thought and emotion.

In his book *Anatomy of an Illness,* Norman Cousins described his experience with rheumatoid arthritis, a classic autoimmune disorder. He was getting progressively worse when he decided to intervene on his own behalf, so to speak. He recalled the work of Walter B. Cannon on the wisdom of the body and particularly the observations of Hans Selye that emotional factors such as frustration or suppressed rage could lead to adrenal exhaustion, which, we know from modern research, can markedly impair immune function. Cousins cured himself through the application of what he called "positive emotions," to counteract the effect of "negative emotions." He also credited high doses of Vitamin C for his recovery, but admitted that this might have been the result of a placebo effect.

Cousins's book and an article he wrote for the *New England Journal of Medicine* made a strong impression on both the general public and doctors at the time. The movement to seek out practitioners of alternative methods of treatment had already begun. Historically, many doctors knew of the power of the mind. Cousins must have been preaching to the converted, however, for most of medicine has continued to follow the mechanistic approach to diagnosis and treatment that he so eloquently decried. Mainstream medicine has not yet realized that the movement to alternative medicine in the United States reflects the failure of conventional medicine to deal effectively with a variety of ills, the pain syndromes representing the best example.

It may perhaps be taken as a faint sign of hope that an article and editorial appeared in the *Journal of the American Medical Association* in April 1999 on the physical benefit of writing about stressful experiences in patients with rheumatoid arthritis and asthma. This study is similar to the one reported on page 119, in which writing about emotionally disturbing situations produced a drop in Epstein-Barr antibody titers. According to our classification, asthma is an equivalent of TMS, but rheumatoid arthritis, which is an autoimmune disorder, is not. This is further evidence that emotional factors play a role in the etiology of autoimmune disorders. That the study warranted an editorial titled "Emotional Expression and Disease Outcome" is a basis for guarded optimism that American medicine is beginning to become aware of the relationship between emotions and physical illness.

Cardiovascular Disorders

Hypertension

Although I have had a few patients who developed high blood pressure after their pain went away, it was not included as an equivalent of TMS for a number of reasons.

First, it is a disorder without symptoms. People don't know they have hypertension, except in rare instances, until their blood pressures are taken. So no distraction, no avoidance strategy is at work.

Second, hypertension can contribute to such serious medical problems as atherosclerosis (hardening of the arteries) and enlargement of the heart, putting it into a category different from TMS and its equivalents.

Finally, some cases of hypertension are thought by the experts to be genetic, which is not true of TMS or any of its equivalents, and still others are due to very specific disorders such as kidney disease or an adrenal tumor known as pheochromocytoma.

Even though it is not a TMS equivalent, there is evidence that some hypertension is a psychogenic disorder. At the Cardiovascular Center of the New York Hospital–Cornell Medical College an internist, Samuel J. Mann, has concluded that repressed emotions and *not* "consciously perceived and reported stress" play the primary role in the development of many cases of hypertension. His findings are very exciting; they represent a breakthrough in the field of "physical" medicine. Ultimately, physical doctors like Dr. Mann and me must recognize the psychogenic nature of physical disorders, for physical symptoms are our domain, not the psychiatrist's. The people psychiatrists see represent only a small proportion of the psychosomatic population—which is beginning to look as though it includes everyone.

Another group of investigators headed by Dr. Peter Schnall of the same center demonstrated conclusively that hypertension was related to "job strain" at work, and identified lack of control as an important specific factor. It is not difficult to imagine that this lack of control translated into unconscious rage that could not be expressed for obvious reasons and was automatically repressed.

Hypertension is a condition that appears to be more serious than TMS and its equivalents but not as serious as other cardiovascular conditions, the autoimmune diseases or cancer. Psychologically, one would hypothesize that the need for physical pathology is greater in hypertensives than in TMS patients but not as great as those who develop more serious diseases. I will state more than once that this may be related to the magnitude of the rage and the depth of repression. The more deeply repressed the rage, the greater the potential for a serious illness. That idea is, of course, highly theoretical.

Arteriosclerosis, Atherosclerosis, Hardening of the Arteries

These are all designations for the buildup of fatty deposits (plaques) on the inner surface of arteries, resulting in narrowing and leading to the possibility of blockage. In the brain the result may be a stroke; in the heart these may be a variety of reactions, including a myocardial infarction (heart attack). Arteries anywhere in the body can be affected, resulting in such diverse problems as circulatory disorders in the legs, kidney disease or blindness.

Whether or not and how rapidly arteriosclerosis proceeds depends on several factors, including heredity, predisposition, diet, the presence of diabetes, amount of exercise and emotions.

Drs. Meyer Friedman and Ray Rosenman, in their book *Type A Behavior and Your Heart,* suggested that psychological factors might play a role in the development of coronary artery atherosclerosis. It is now almost part of the culture to categorize some people as type A. The book suggests that to be hard-driving, workaholic, aggressive, competitive, hostile—the attributes of the Type A personality—somehow predispose to coronary arteriosclerosis. Further research suggests that hostility is the most important of these personality characteristics. Since hostility *may be* the outward manifestation of internal rage, it is reasonable to consider that rage is the leading causative factor. The Type A personality traits are similar to those that lead to TMS and its equivalents.

A study published in 1990 gave further support to the importance of emotional factors in the development of coronary artery atherosclerosis. Dean Ornish and his colleagues at the University of California School of Medicine demonstrated that arteriosclerotic plaques in the coronary arteries could actually be diminished over a period of months if patients adhered to a program consisting of a special diet; stress management activities like meditation, relaxation, imagery and breathing techniques; moderate aerobic exercise; and group discussions for social support and encouragement to maintain the program. Control patients showed a gradual increase in atherosclerosis while study patients had fewer episodes of cardiac angina (pain) and reduced hardening in their coronary arteries. It is my view that attention to psychological factors was the primary reason for the reduction in coronary atherosclerosis.

If emotional factors are a leading cause of arteriosclerosis in coronary arteries, it is logical to conclude that they play a role in atherosclerosis everywhere in the body.

Mitral Valve Prolapse

This is an interesting, mysterious structural abnormality in one of the heart valves. It appears to be harmless, since it does not impede normal cardiac function. Varying in severity from year to year, in some people it disappears entirely.

Research has found that the condition seems to be the result of autonomic nervous system activity, like TMS and many of its equivalents. An unsigned editorial in *Lancet* on

October 3, 1987, reviewed the medical literature linking the sympathetic nervous system to MVP and noted that similar autonomic dysfunction is found in people with anxiety. I believe that the chemical changes that have been associated with both anxiety and MVP are the result of unconscious emotional phenomena, that repressed rage may be the common denominator in these seemingly disparate medical conditions. Once more, psychology drives the chemistry and not vice versa.

Another study notes the high incidence of MVP in patients with fibromyalgia, which is part of TMS.

In my experience MVP is not the cause of cardiac rhythm irregularities, as is generally assumed. They are both psychosomatic and, therefore, may coexist. People with MVP may go for long periods without irregular heartbeats while the mitral valve prolapse is constantly there.

Cancer

Many studies and observations through the years have suggested the possible role of emotions in the etiology and course of cancer. For anyone interested in this subject I suggest reading the work of Lawrence LeShan, Kenneth Pelletier, Carl Simonton, Steven Locke and Lydia Temoshok. Dr. Locke's book *The Healer Within* (written with Douglas Colligan) has an excellent review of the work that has been done in this field over the years.

There is ample evidence that psychological factors play some role in the genesis and the subsequent course of cancer once it has begun. Precisely what that role is has yet to be determined.

All human beings probably generate new growths regularly but the immune system recognizes them as undesirable entities and promptly destroys them. Do emotions participate in that earliest stage of carcinogenesis when the new growths represent only a few malignant cells? That is a question that should be addressed by cancer research.

Should the immune system fail in that first mission, cancer cells continue to reproduce themselves and the tumor grows. Can emotions play a role in this second stage? In the chapter on cancer and the mind in their book *The Healer Within,* Locke and Colligan described the research of Lydia Temoshok on patients with malignant melanoma. She and her colleagues found that most of these patients had strong needs to be nice. They never expressed anger, fear or sadness and they tended to worry about their loved ones rather than themselves. Bad feelings were not allowed. How interesting, I thought, that many patients with TMS have the same personality traits. Why did they get TMS instead of malignant melanoma?

The theory I propose is that beneath some cancer patients' nice exterior is a monumental rage that is both the result of the compulsion to be a good person (goodism) and the source of that need. As stated in Part I of this book, the compulsion to please is enraging to the narcissistic inner self and at the same time the parent in the mind is saying, "You are such a nasty, angry person inside. You had better be nice." We must accustom ourselves to the idea that the brain-mind is a conglomeration of thoughts and feelings that are often at odds with each other. It is not the neat, well-organized, logical organ we would like it to be.

Other psychological factors have been related to cancer. Psychologists have associated it with melancholia and depression for years. Traumatic life events are often precursors of cancer. Some cancer patients are emotionally restrained, others feel hopeless and helpless, and many have a history of poor relationships with parents. All of these have been observed as well in patients with TMS and its equivalents. Again, why do TMS patients get a basically benign process instead of cancer?

Essential to TMS theory is that many aspects of life are sources of pressure, as described in Part I of this book, and that these pressures induce internal rage. The psychodynamic interaction of perfectionism, goodism and rage is an example. Stressful life events are enraging in the unconscious; the poor parenting and abuses of infancy and childhood sometimes result in permanent rage.

Whether the accumulated rage results in TMS and its equivalents, autoimmune disease, cardiovascular disorders or cancer may be a function of the magnitude of the rage and the depth or power of its repression, according to TMS theory. People who suffer great personal losses like the death of a parent or spouse upon whom they depended emotionally may generate enormous amounts of rage, enough to bring on cancer. The reason many psychological factors have been related to cancer is that they all induce internal rage. In my view, that is the common denominator that leads to a variety of psychosomatic reactions, some benign, some malignant. Obviously, if one is to employ psychotherapy in an effort to reverse a psychosomatic process, work must be done on the sources of the rage, not the rage itself.

My experience with TMS has given me a unique opportunity to theorize on the subject. I have dealt successfully with a disorder that in most cases is clearly the result of repressed rage and have done so by teaching patients to acknowledge that fact and, if necessary, work with a psychotherapist. As will be seen in Part III of this book, 85 to 90 percent of patients will be successful without psychotherapy. Whether my program would be applicable to people with autoimmune, cardiovascular or cancerous diseases awaits study. The principle might apply, but I suspect that the therapeutic process would be much more arduous with these more serious disorders than with TMS.

This brings to mind one of the more recent miracle cancer cures originally reported in *Vogue*. Alice Epstein was diagnosed with a very malignant kidney cancer and was told that she did not have long to live. She rejected that prognosis, began to take a close look at her life and began psychotherapy. She survived and has shared that experience in a book.

Norman Cousins and others have been discussing this process for years.

There are many questions to be answered, mysteries to be solved in the realm of mindbody medicine. For example, what determines whether the brain will choose cancer or cardiovascular or autoimmune disease when the rage is more deeply hidden? It will prove easier to identify the pathophysiological processes involved in each case than to determine why cancer, why rheumatoid arthritis or coronary artery disease.

Homo sapiens represents the ultimate in evolution, at least in this solar system. The crowning glory of our species is the mind, no doubt still evolving, but already quite remarkable. The power of speech and creative thought, to take only two of its abilities, are so special and intricate that we still have no notion of how they are accomplished.

The study of emotions is also in its infancy, to such an extent that many medical scientists are not yet aware of the impact of emotions on bodily function. It is the purpose of this book to draw attention to that connection.

PART THREE

The Treatment of Mindbody Disorders

9

The Therapeutic Program:
The Power of Knowledge

Since you are reading this book, chances are you have suffered a pain syndrome for weeks, months or years. The length of time is not important for the TMS diagnosis, nor is the fact that you may have had recurrent episodes of pain that began with a physical incident or injury.

Consider this your initial consultation with me. Your pain may be in the low back, accompanied by numbness, tingling or weakness in any part of one or both legs. It may be in the middle or upper back. Or it may be in the neck and shoulder, with pain, numbness, tingling or weakness in one or both arms and hands. It may be in the shoulder joint region, the elbow, the wrist, the fingers, the hip area, the knee, the ankle, the top or bottom of the foot, on one or both sides.

All of these are common manifestations of TMS.

The pain may be worse during the day or at night. It may be severe when you first awaken and try to get out of bed, gradually improving as the day goes on; or you may be at your best when you get up in the morning and suffer increasing pain in the course of the day. It may be aggravated or improved by sitting, standing in one place or walking. You may be afraid to bend or lift; if you can't do those things you will not be able to do your job, run or engage in any sport or exercise. You may be afraid to do anything physical, no matter how easy the task or maneuver.

Or you may have continued to be physically active, including participating in vigorous sports, in spite of the pain. You may get pain at strange, illogical times and not get it when it seems you should.

These are all common scenarios for people with TMS and are classic examples of how they become programmed to have pain at certain times and in association with many different activities or physical postures.

Most of the time you are under the impression that something is wrong with your back or neck or shoulders, a structural defect, deterioration or degeneration of parts of your spine, a bulging or herniated disc, fibromyalgia, a tear or strain in a muscle, tendonitis somewhere. These diagnoses are usually supported by X rays, a CT scan or MRI studies, and it is highly likely that your pain got considerably worse when you learned what these tests showed.

Your life may be literally dominated by the pain syndrome; it haunts your waking hours. You have been to many doctors and tried many treatments, but, though it is sometimes better for a while, the condition invariably returns.

Your family and friends are sympathetic and constantly warn you to be careful.

I have learned all these things from you in the course of taking your history. The physical examination disclosed either no objective neurological abnormalities or a variety of relatively minor ones like the loss of a tendon reflex, some mild weakness or change in the perception of a painful stimulus like a pinprick. Some of you had extremely limited ability to move around, maneuver on the examination table or bend over, and others were remarkably agile. Virtually all of you, however, experienced pain when I pressed on certain muscles in the lateral buttock, the small of the back and the top of the shoulders. Additionally, about 80 percent of you felt pain when I pressed on the long tendons on the side of both thighs.

Because of the physical findings and the history, I concluded that you had TMS and proceeded to tell you what that meant. I said that the structural abnormalities previously identified were not the cause of your pain and that I would present evidence then and in the course of my lectures to buttress that conclusion. The pain, stiffness, burning, pressure, numbness, tingling and weakness were caused by mild oxygen deprivation in the muscles, nerves or tendons involved in each case. In itself this was harmless. Although it could produce more severe pain than anything else I knew of in clinical medicine, you would not be left with residual damage when your symptoms disappeared.

I then proceeded to explain why the brain had seen fit to reduce the blood flow to these areas, causing the distressing symptoms; how the rage and other powerful feelings in the unconscious were threatening to break out into consciousness, and the pain had to be created as a distraction to prevent that from happening. In most cases you were aware of the important psychological factors, like the stresses in your life, perfectionism and goodism or childhood trauma, that were responsible for your pain. You were reassured that resolution (cure) would come with understanding of the process. I said that all of this would be amplified and clarified in the course of two basic lectures, since there was not enough time to present the entire story during an office consultation. We will have spent forty-five minutes together.

This digest of the initial consultation suggests what the therapeutic program will be. We must somehow thwart the brain's strategy. To accomplish that I encourage patients to:

> Repudiate the structural diagnosis, the "physical" reason for the pain (TMS is a different kind of physical process)
> Acknowledge the psychological basis for the pain

➤ Accept the psychological explanation and all of its ramifications as normal for healthy people in our society

Repudiate the Structural Diagnosis

The pain will not stop unless you are able to say, "I have a normal back; I now know that the pain is due to a basically harmless condition, initiated by the brain to serve a psychological purpose, and that the structural abnormalities that have been found on X ray, CT scan or MRI are normal changes associated with activity and aging."

This initial realization is essential to thwart the brain's strategy, which is to keep your attention firmly fixed on your body and unaware of the threatening feelings in your unconscious. As I explained in Part I of this book, the mind fears that the unconscious rage will break out into the consciousness.

Why should you dismiss the significance of structural abnormalities? In most cases the abnormality does not adequately explain the pain; it is often in the wrong place and the pain may occur at the wrong time, such as when you are resting comfortably in bed. I recall a man who loaded his truck all day long and had pain only when he bent over the sink to shave in the morning. Perhaps most convincing is that I have seen thousands of people with a large variety of structural changes in their spines (or who had a diagnosis like fibromyalgia) recover completely days or weeks after learning about TMS. Experience is a great, if difficult, teacher.

The Principle of Simultaneity

TMS symptoms often begin in association with a known structural abnormality—for example, back and leg pain in someone whose CT scan or MRI demonstrates a herniated disc in roughly the right location to explain the symptoms. In these cases the speed with which the person becomes free of pain tells us that the disc herniation was not responsible for the pain.

The presence of a disc abnormality is a stumbling block to many patients who are not aware that this is a demonstration of the cleverness and ingenuity of the mind when it wishes to create a physical distraction. The mind is aware of everything that goes on in the body, including the site of herniated discs, meniscus tears in the knee joints, and tears of the rotator cuff at the shoulder. It may sound fanciful, but experience makes it clear that the brain will initiate TMS pain where a structural abnormality exists, the better to impress you and more firmly keep your attention on your body, just as it will induce pain at the site of an old injury.

The tendency to attribute the pain to a structural abnormality is irresistible and in some instances may be legitimate, but in most cases it clearly is not; TMS is usually the true cause of the pain. A doctor familiar with TMS can make the distinction.

Fortunately, new studies are making it easier to convince patients that structural abnormalities are widespread and seldom painful. One of the most impressive appeared in the *New England Journal of Medicine* in July 1994. A group of research workers from the Hoag Memorial Hospital of Newport Beach, California, and the Cleveland Clinic reported finding lumbar disc bulges and protrusions on MRI in sixty-four of ninety-eight men and women who had never had back pain. This is only one of the more recent of many studies through the years documenting that structural abnormalities do not cause back pain. Despite this, almost all physicians and other practitioners continue to attribute pain to structural abnormalities.

Acknowledge the Psychological Basis for the Pain

The brain tries desperately to divert our attention from rage in the unconscious. This is an automatic reaction of the mind, not based on logic or reason. So we must bring reason to the process. This is the heart of the very important concept—that we can influence unconscious, automatic reactions by the application of conscious thought processes. It is no longer a theory, for we have seen it work in thousands of patients.

The many reasons for repressed rage were discussed in Part I of this book. You may want to review them again now. You must think about the rage rather than the "where" and the "how bad" of the pain.

The realm of the unconscious is not logical or reasonable like the conscious mind. It reacts automatically and sometimes in very strange ways. The development of TMS is a good example.

You ask, "What is the sense in producing pain to distract one's attention from repressed rage? I would rather deal with the rage than have the pain."

That's logical. But the way the human emotional system is now organized, in evolutionary terms, dictates how it will react, and it is often not rational. Since the brain is evolving, there may come a time, centuries or millennia from now, when the unconscious will be more rational. But for now we must have a sense of how different the unconscious mind is from the conscious to understand how TMS and its equivalents occur. The unconscious mind is apparently terrified by the rage and reacts accordingly.

Accept the Psychological

We must say to ourselves, "It's all right to be the way we are: illogical, unconsciously enraged, like a child having a temper tantrum. That's part of being human and it is universal."

I have enunciated three principles of treatment: repudiate the physical, acknowledge and accept the psychological. On a practical, day-to-day basis, how can we work toward accomplishing these ends? Following are some strategies.

Think Psychological

I tell my patients that they must consciously think about repressed rage and the reasons for it whenever they are aware of the pain. This is in contradiction to what the brain is trying to do. This effort is a counterattack, an attempt to undo the brain's strategy. It is essential to focus on unpleasant, threatening thoughts and feelings to deny the pain its purpose—to divert your attention from those feelings.

When the pain is severe, it is difficult to concentrate on feelings, but you must regard the process as a contest in which your conscious will is pitted against the unconscious, automatic reactions of the brain.

Talk to Your Brain

It sounds silly, but it's very effective. The conscious mind addresses the unconscious, the more forcefully the better. Successfully treated patients report that when they feel a twinge of pain, the kind of thing that used to be a harbinger of an attack, they talk to or shout at themselves and the pain disappears. You tell your mind that you know what it's doing, that you know the physical pain is harmless and is a distraction from the repressed rage, and that you no longer intend to be diverted and intimidated. You might even tell it to increase the blood flow to the involved tissues. This is particularly reasonable in light of contemporary research that demonstrates how the brain communicates with the rest of the body.

Make a Written List

List all the pressures in your life, since they all contribute to your inner rage. There are self-imposed pressures, typical of the conscientious perfectionist or the goodist, and the pressures of everyday life, including "happy" things like marriage and children, since they, too, represent great pressure. You should also list anger left over from childhood.

Patients have found this to be a very helpful exercise. I recall one man who said he was shocked to see the length of his list.

Patients often ask, "Won't it make things worse if I concentrate on all the troubles and problems in my life?" Paradoxically, no, for it is the failure to realize their impact on the inner mind that leads to such conditions as TMS, heartburn, migraine headache, anxiety and depression. By identifying and dealing with sources of pressure consciously, you reduce their potential negative effect in the unconscious.

A Daily Reflection or Meditation Period

This part of the treatment is essential for very busy people who don't have a moment to think of anything but their work during the day. The treatment for TMS and its equivalents is to think your way out of it. This is best done in quiet and solitude, so a time must be found each day when you can sit and think about what it takes to get better.

Physical Activity and the Fear Factor

We know that the purpose of physical symptoms like TMS and its equivalents is to keep attention focused on the body. If the pain disappears but you are still fearful of physical activity, recurrent pain, injury and progressive degeneration of spinal elements, the battle has not yet been won. The pain will return unless you overcome those fears. So patients are advised to resume normal, unrestricted physical activity once the pain is gone, or nearly so, and when they feel confidence in the diagnosis. Patients have reported that becoming active may take months, which is not difficult to understand considering their years of exposure to misconceptions about the presumed fragility of the back.

Never do this or that, do it this way, we're told; be careful, you'll hurt yourself; your spine is out of line; the discs are degenerated and the spinal bones are rubbing together; one of your legs is shorter than the other; people weren't meant to walk upright; you've got flat feet; don't swim the crawl or the breast stroke; don't arch your back; never sleep on your stomach; always bend your knees when you bend at the waist or come back up; don't lift; don't do sit-ups, do crunches; and on and on.

All of these admonitions and prohibitions, enhanced by poor medical advice, keep your attention riveted on your body, which is your brain's intention.

The path to resumption of full physical activity, without fear, may be slow and uneven. Don't worry if you begin to exercise too soon and experience some pain. You cannot hurt yourself; TMS is a benign process. Continuing pain with activity means the brain is still in the process of changing its programming. You must bide your time, try and try again, and stay secure in the knowledge that you will prevail in the end. This has proven to be the case for thousands of patients.

On the other hand, don't start the physical program too soon—not because of potential physical harm, but because the brain may still be programmed in the TMS mode. I recommend waiting a few weeks after you accept the TMS diagnosis so the pain can diminish, confidence can be strengthened, and the brain will have had time to be reprogrammed.

Prevention, Not Aspirin

The goal of treatment is to change the unconscious mind's reaction to emotional states. When this has been accomplished, pain will cease. Since the therapeutic process takes time, you must look on it as an exercise in preventive medicine. In a sense we are stopping tomorrow's pain and any pain that might occur thereafter. This is different from the conventional concept, which is to treat the pain. Merely dealing with pain is analogous to treating fever instead of the infection that causes it. We seek to eliminate the cause of the pain, which is why I say knowledge is the penicillin in the treatment of TMS. However, unlike antibiotics, the use of knowledge to reverse the process usually takes time. You must be patient—but persistent. In most cases the cessation of pain takes only a few weeks, although banishing the fear may take a lot longer.

How the Strategy Works

Why does repudiating the physical and acknowledging and accepting the psychological make the pain stop?

Remember that the purpose of the pain is to divert attention from what's going on emotionally and to keep you focused on the body. In essence it is a contest for conscious attention.

Recall what happened to Helen, whom I wrote about in Chapter 1. When both the process of repression and the strategy of distraction with pain failed, her powerful emotions exploded into consciousness. Her attention was now on the emotions that had become conscious. Clearly she had no need for the pain, so it disappeared immediately.

Since we cannot re-create Helen's experience in everyone, we do the next best thing—getting you to focus on the unconscious rage, imagining and visualizing it, and thinking about all the pressures that produced it. Reflection is a therapeutic tool. For most patients it will banish the pain and usually prevent its return. For most people just thinking about the rage in this fashion is as good as experiencing it.

I wish I could say that I had devised this strategy through brilliant thinking. The truth is that I discovered it by accident. Long before I understood the details of the psychological genesis of the pain of TMS, I had observed that a few patients got better after merely being told that the pain was of psychological rather than structural origin. I puzzled over that mystery for many years before I realized that the role of the pain was to divert attention from frightening feelings.

Knowledge Is the Cure

For some people simply shifting attention from the physical to the psychological will do the trick. Others need more information on how the strategy works, and still others require psychotherapy. But in every case knowledge is essential to the "cure," for by making people aware of what is going on both physically and psychologically we frustrate the brain's strategy. (I'm enclosing the word *cure* in quotation marks to remind the reader that TMS is not a disease: A person gets better and banishes the pain—but there is really nothing to "cure.") By changing the focus of attention from the body to the psyche we render the pain useless, take away its purpose and reveal what it was trying to hide. In a small number of cases the person must actually experience the emotion, like rage or profound sadness, before the pain will cease. This always requires the help of a properly trained psychotherapist.

I recall a patient in his fifties who carried a lifelong anger at his mother, of which he was somewhat aware. However, his pain persisted until he was able, in the course of therapy with a psychologist, to experience his repressed rage.

Book Cures

As evidence of the critical role of knowledge, many people have reported success in banishing the pain simply from studying my books on TMS, particularly the more recent one, *Healing Back Pain*. Consider the following excerpt from a letter from James Campobello dated November 13, 1991. It is reprinted with his permission:

> I'm writing to thank you for what you have done for me. Specifically, your book *Healing Back Pain* saved me from a life of disability.
>
> I'm forty-three years old and, until my back problem, I had never had any serious injury or illness. In March of 1989 I gradually developed back trouble. It started out as a slightly stiff lower back, and by the end of a week I was in severe, debilitating pain with continuous spasms.
>
> For two years I suffered from nearly constant back pain. It ranged from mild to severe, but it never left completely. Without going into all the dreadful details, it was miserable. I couldn't sit for more than a half hour, I couldn't bend, I couldn't lift, I couldn't ride a bike for more than two minutes. I had given up almost all the activities I enjoy. I worked standing up, rested frequently by lying on a desk, and spent my free time lying on my family-room floor.
>
> I went through the gamut of the medical (and pseudo-medical) professions, to no avail. I saw five different physicians, including the top back specialists in the area. I went through three different therapy programs, with five different therapists. I tried yoga, acupuncture, and chiropractics. Nothing helped; whenever I made a small improvement, soon afterward I had a setback.

However, after reading (and rereading) your book and applying its approach, my back went from disabled to normal in about two months. I am now doing everything I used to do—sitting normally, bike-riding, driving for hours, playing sports, bending and lifting like a normal person—things that I thought I had given up for good. I have been completely healthy for over six months now.

I was skeptical, to say the least, when I was first given your book. I almost didn't finish reading it, because your theory just didn't seem credible. However, the personality type did sound a lot like me, so I finished the book (but remained a skeptic).

My girlfriend, who was the one who found the book and bought it for me, read it a week later and urged me to read it again. (Actually she said something like, "If you don't see yourself on every page of that book then you're either crazy or blind. Read it again.") Out of desperation, plus a grudging acknowledgment that the basic concept might fit me, I did so.

I started improving gradually but steadily. At that point I called to make an appointment with you in hopes of completing the cure through your lecture-group treatment. However, in the month before my appointment, I reread the book four more times, continued to apply your approach, and continued to improve. When the time neared for my appointment, I found I didn't need it. By the end of six weeks I was basically healthy. During that time I stopped the physical therapy, visits to the chiropractor, pills, stretching and back exercises. I haven't done (or avoided) any special back activities in the time since then—almost eight months—and I feel fine.

If I had not been through it myself, I wouldn't believe it. My problem seemed like structural defects in my back. I had been diagnosed as having a variety of bone and disc problems, and I was on the verge of disc removal and bone fusion surgery. (I can't tell you how grateful I am that you saved me from that!)

Mr. Campobello has corresponded with me since that original letter and continues to be free of pain or restriction.

Recently he enclosed a copy of a therapeutic regimen he designed for a friend. I have entitled it Jim Campobello's Therapeutic Program for Overcoming TMS:

First, you must decide that you will make a serious attempt at Dr. Sarno's technique. The technique only works for people who make a strong effort to apply it. You must either believe that it can work for you, or you must be so desperate that you will try very hard to do it even if you don't believe in it.

I did not believe in it when I first read the book. My nature is very skeptical; I didn't believe in mental powers of any kind, and I had given up on the miracles. However, I was desperate. I was in constant pain. My life consisted of standing up to do what little work I could, and lying on a mat on the floor at home the rest of the day. So even though I didn't think it could help, my wife convinced me to try it. You can do the same thing.

So first you must make a commitment to try the book's approach. It costs nothing, but you must be willing to spend some time on it every day for at least a month. You might as well try—what have you got to lose?

I don't think there is one exact way to do it, but I will tell you what worked for me and recommend that you try it.

1. Read about 30 pages of the book every day. Don't just go over the words—think about them! Pay

attention to what he says, and think about how it applies to you. It's very easy to be inattentive, so force yourself to concentrate on the ideas. When you see parts that remind you of yourself, be especially attentive. Also, keep reminding yourself that the people described in the book had problems similar to yours, and they were cured. When you finish reading the book, start it again the next day. You must read it continuously for a month or more. And you must pay attention every time you read it.

2. Set aside time every day to think about what problems might be bothering you, what might be in your life and in your mind that is causing your back trouble. Spend at least 30 minutes every day thinking about this. I used to take 15 minutes in the morning, when I first got up, and then 30 minutes in the evening. Use this time for the following:

Think about everything that might possibly bother you—work or school pressure, family responsibility, financial matters, etc. Be as specific as possible. You cannot simply say, "I'm worried about work"—that isn't enough. You must try to identify every specific item you can think of. I found it useful to write lists to keep track of it. (When you are very specific you can think of quite a few things.) Pay attention to all areas of your life, big and little. Consider not only the obvious problems, but try to speculate about hidden things too. Consider both the real and imagined things that might be troubling you.

Once you have identified your problems, divide them into two categories: those that you can do something about, and those that are beyond your control. Be realistic about where each one fits. The ones you can do something about, start taking action on. Do whatever you can to correct them, or try to at least. The ones you have no control over, tell yourself that you know they bother you, but you must accept them—and most important, you will not let them cause you any more back pain. Remember, you don't have to eliminate your problems for the cure to work, you just have to be aware of the process.

Think about what you are like—what is it in you that lets these problems create such pain. I am a typical Sarno type—perfectionist, easily angered, highly motivated, high achiever, somewhat compulsive and impatient with other people. Those are the part of my personality that led my mind to develop back pain. However, there are other types that get it. One of my co-workers is a happy, easygoing, very pleasant woman, but she got back pain as bad as mine, and the book cured her, too. (It took her about three months, by the way, but she is perfectly healthy now.) Try to learn what is inside you that needs that distraction. What permits the pain to develop and persist? Be honest about yourself. Again, remember that you don't have to change your personality for the cure to work—you just have to understand and fight it.

3. All day long, keep reminding yourself of the whole process. Whenever a problem occurs, think, "Okay, I don't like that, but I'm not going to let it go to my back and cause pain." Whenever you feel back pain (or if you are like I was and it hurts all the time, whenever it feels especially bad), think, "My back is acting up. What is going on in my life or in my mind to make it hurt?"

4. After you have worked on the above for three or four weeks, start to take small steps to test your progress. Don't do too much too soon. Just look for tiny improvements, find something you can do that doesn't

hurt quite as much as it used to. Go very slowly, but after a few more weeks you will notice your back is a little better. Build on the small steps—the slightest improvement is a sign that the process is working, and that should encourage you to stick with it.

5. Don't give up. Believe me, I know how depressing and discouraging it is. Yet there is hope. But in order for it to work, you must put in the time and effort to make it work.

I inserted an addition into Mr. Campobello's program stating that goodism is just as potent an instigator of unconscious rage as perfectionism, as is the anger that goes back to childhood experiences, which is very important for some people with TMS.

The Placebo and the Nocebo

An excellent article published in the *Journal of the American Medical Association* in 1994 pointed out the necessity of looking very critically at the results of any treatment because of a possible placebo effect. If someone believes that a preferred treatment is good—though it may be of no value, like a sugar pill—relief of symptoms and even cure may result. The effect is based on blind faith. Unfortunately, the effect is invariably temporary and symptoms soon return. This is why the many treatments employed for back pain, including physical therapy, medication and surgery, ultimately fail; their temporary benefits are attributable to the placebo phenomenon.

I refer to it as the "magnificent placebo" because it demonstrates the great power of the mind to alter bodily function. Placebos have been known to temporarily reverse cancer.

What of people who have surgery and remain symptom-free for long periods? Since the purpose of symptoms is to distract from what is occurring in the unconscious, if pain is relieved by the placebo effect of a powerful treatment like surgery, the brain will simply move the pain to another location or even to another organ of the body so that the distraction can continue.

One of my patients gave a history of having had successful low back surgery, whereupon he began to have persistent stomach ulcer problems. This continued for years, despite treatment, but when it finally came under control he began to have severe neck pain. At that point he entered my program and did very well once the TMS diagnosis was made.

Many patients, however, have recurrences at the site of surgery when the surgery has functioned as a placebo.

Why Treatment for TMS Is Not a Placebo

TMS treatment is primarily a process of education; blind faith is not involved. Patients must conclude that what they hear is logical and reasonable, satisfying themselves that the disorder described as TMS pertains to them.

The therapeutic result is almost always permanent.

The fact that large numbers of people are "cured" by reading books about TMS is certainly not a placebo. There is no treatment, no interaction with a "healer"—only the acquisition of information. It is the knowledge that gets the job done.

Recently we have begun to hear of the *nocebo,* the reverse phenomenon in which people may get sick from "bad" interactions. The word means "I will harm." Those who know about voodoo practices are aware of its existence. An old family physician I know had a patient who decided she was going to die and promptly did so though nothing was wrong with her.

The pain epidemic that plagues Western society today is almost entirely a result of the nocebo. You have an attack of back and leg pain, visit the doctor and are told that it is probably a problem with the spine, most likely a herniated disc. Though TMS is harmless, being told that the pain is the direct result of a structural problem ensures that the pain will continue. Advised to stay in bed, you believe it must be serious, and the pain worsens. Despite bed rest the pain continues and an MRI is ordered; not only does it show a herniated disc at L5–S1, but the doctor informs you that the two discs above the herniated one are degenerated and the vertebral bodies are rubbing together. This is terrible; you now have objective evidence that you have a "bad" back. Often immediate surgery is recommended, or you are told it may be necessary if you do not respond to conservative treatment. The result: intensifying pain.

I have heard this history thousands of times. When finally I see the patients, they have tried every known treatment, or have had surgery, sometimes twice, for the nocebo effect has been nurtured throughout. Regardless of the treatment employed, it is always based on structural or muscle deficiency pathology, which deepens your fear and enhances the persistence of pain.

Is it any wonder that some people can get better reading a book that explains the true reason for the pain and tells them that in reality they have normal backs, that most herniated discs are normal abnormalities? That is reversing the nocebo, not by placebo, but by enlisting the power of the mind to heal the body. More specifically, TMS is "cured" by teaching people to be aware of the nature of the mind-body connection. Following Dr. Pert's suggestion, mind and body should no longer be hyphenated. It is one word, as the title of this book implies.

The Program

It begins in my office with a consultation. This, I often tell patients, is your first lesson. They are then scheduled to attend two lectures: the first on the anatomy and physiology of TMS, and diagnostic issues; the second on the psychology and treatment of TMS. The material in this book is covered in those lectures. Some have referred to the program as a talking cure, which is certainly unique in the treatment of a physical disorder.

The consultation and lectures bring about disappearance of symptoms in 80 to 85 percent of patients, usually within a matter of weeks. Those who continue to have significant pain are invited to attend weekly meetings at which the cardinal features of TMS and the principles and practice of treatment are reviewed. People often say they must hear some things repeatedly before they sink in. Sometimes something is said that rings a bell or has special meaning for the person. We discuss various problems and pitfalls in the recovery process, and patients are encouraged to talk about their specific situations.

If pain persists despite the lectures and group meetings, it means that deeper exploration is necessary and psychotherapy is prescribed. This is successful in most cases, leaving us with only about 5 percent of patients overall who continue to have significant pain.

What makes the treatment effective? I have said that awareness is the principal therapeutic ingredient. Undoubtedly other factors are at work. In Part I of this book I introduced the concepts of Heinz Kohut, who believed that narcissistic rage was the cause of certain emotional disorders. I am suggesting that we all generate narcissistic rage (to a greater or lesser extent), which is why psychosomatic disorders are universal in Western society, varying only in type and severity.

It was a patient, Muriel Campbell, who introduced me to

Kohut's work. She had this to say about why my program is effective:

> Since patients with TMS are in a state of rage, they must have been narcissistically injured. Expressing the rage somatically, they visit a traditional physician who advises bed rest or surgery, therefore further narcissistically injuring and disempowering them, therefore, increasing the rage. Feeling helpless, they climb into bed, and as you have described so vividly, they feel further narcissistically injured and powerless. However, unlike the unempathic parents, when they finally visit you, you empathically welcome and affirm, as well as calm and soothe, these feelings of rage. You also offer an experience of essential alikeness, by introducing them to other sufferers of TMS. In this manner you not only make them aware of these disavowed aspects of rage, but effectively diminish it. You activate a sense of power (grandiose self) after that sense has been injured and depleted. You can do it quickly, because rage is not viewed as a drive, but rather a disintegration product following a narcissistic injury, which your empathy diminishes by providing the selfobject functions of affirming (mirroring), calming and soothing (idealization), and essential alikeness (twinship). The patient is of course vulnerable to further injury, and rage, which explains why some of us return.

I agree with some of this interpretation of the effectiveness of my therapeutic program, since it is clear that there is something at work besides the knowledge imparted, which I consider the most important ingredient. It may very well be that mirroring, idealization and twinship are at work. If so there may be a reduction in internal anger, which is certainly compatible with the disappearance of pain. This may be the reason patients frequently report that the lectures were very important in their recovery, providing them with something they did not get from reading the books on TMS.

However, according to TMS theory pain is not a somatic expression of rage, as Ms. Campbell stated, nor do I consider rage a "disintegration product." Rather, as has been said repeatedly, it is a reaction to internal and external pressures.

The problem with the pure Kohutian interpretation of the efficacy of my therapeutic program (used by Ms. Campbell) is that my patients are not aware that they are in a rage because it is unconscious. Being made aware of the existence of unconscious rage and the reasons for it is the primary therapeutic ingredient.

On the other hand, one of Ms. Campbell's points should be emphasized. People who have recurrent attacks of pain over many years must surely feel out of control, and that must be enraging to the inner self. They never know when the next attack will come or how severe it will be. They are totally or partially restricted in physical activities and find it difficult to plan ahead because of the uncertainty of how their backs will be.

When patients learn that they can actually take control to rid themselves of this terrible scourge, the sense of power may be intoxicating. One woman said that now that she had banished her back pain she felt she could do almost anything with her body. Empowerment is strong medicine.

Pitfalls, Problems, Questions

What You Don't Need to Do to Get Better

Once patients learn that rage is the culprit in TMS and that it has its sources in childhood trauma, the need to be perfect and good and a host of everyday life pressures, they assume that all these stressors must be removed if they are to get better. Logic suggests that if rage is the cause, like the devil, it must be exorcised. If rage could escape from the unconscious and be expressed, as in Helen's case, that would certainly effect a "cure." Unfortunately, that is rarely possible. The rage is repressed, we do not feel it and, therefore, we cannot deal with it.

Nor is it possible for us to change our personalities and stop trying to be perfect and good. If we are aware that we possess these traits we can modify our behavior and lessen whatever negative effects they have on us, but basically we remain the same people we have always been. Even in psychoanalysis, a process that plumbs the emotional depths of a person's psyche, his or her personality does not change. The better we know ourselves, the less feelings like rage will frighten us. Although rage never goes away and we continue to generate it, once we acknowledge it, the rage becomes less threatening, losing some of its sting.

Lifestyle, too, can only rarely undergo substantial change. Fortunately, experience has demonstrated that it is knowledge, not change, that produces the cure. This requires repetition in the learning process.

The Time Factor

We know that psychosomatic processes are not intrinsic to the personality because even pain syndromes that have been present for years may stop in days or weeks. Jim Campobello's experience is typical.

That the pain disappears at all is remarkable and suggests that TMS is a reaction strategy, chosen by the mind because of its effectiveness. Happily, TMS is clearly susceptible to reversal. If the process were personality-bound it would take years to reverse, if that could be accomplished at all.

Most of the people who participate in my program, regardless of how long they have had pain, are free of pain in weeks, although overcoming the fear of physical activity may take longer. What determines the time factor?

Understanding and accepting the nature of TMS is an intellectual process, a function of the conscious mind. Because TMS originates in the unconscious, the new ideas must penetrate and be accepted there for the pain to cease. That's the rub. If the emotions are frightening enough, the mind will be loath to relinquish a strategy that keeps them hidden and impotent. The quality and quantity of the underlying emotion determines how long resolution will take, or whether it will occur at all. Indeed, inability to repudiate the structural explanation for the pain is a measure of the same thing; denial of the syndrome is intrinsic to the syndrome. The mind has decided it cannot do without the pain.

Does that mean we are defeated? Not at all. Sometimes repetition of the principles for a few weeks will do it. If not, there is psychotherapy.

Psychotherapy

Someday we will realize that the study of our personalities is more important than reading, writing and arithmetic. It will be part of basic education to know about the unconscious and repression, most particularly about what each of us is keeping in check. We will learn that a parent, an adult, and a child reside in our brains and that they are often at odds with one another. Psychoeducation will be a prerequisite to holding public office or being in law enforcement, for the better these people know themselves, the better they can serve the public. When I refer someone for psychotherapy I feel as though I am sending them to a special kind of graduate school.

There are two major fields of psychotherapy: behavioral

and insight-oriented (analytical). Behavioral psychotherapy tends to focus on life events and how best to deal with them. Behavioral therapists help people get over phobias like fear of flying, and stop undesirable habits like smoking.

It should be clear from the theories propounded in this book that insight-oriented therapy is the choice for people with TMS or its equivalents. The therapists to whom I refer patients are trained to help them explore the unconscious and become aware of feelings that are buried there, usually because they are frightening, embarrassing or in some way unacceptable. These feelings, and the rage to which they often give rise, are responsible for the many mindbody symptoms I have described. When we become aware of these feelings, in some cases by gradually becoming able to feel them, the physical symptoms become unnecessary and go away.

Psychotherapists often report, "He doesn't even talk about pain anymore, we're so involved in resolving his deep inner conflicts about his marriage"—or about some other emotional issue.

Psychotherapy is a slow process; it is not a quick fix. Because it deals with issues that affect virtually all aspects of our lives, time devoted to the process is well spent, no matter how long it may be.

One great drawback to psychotherapy is cost. This is becoming an increasing problem as managed health care providers show growing reluctance to reimburse for psychotherapy. This trend reflects a sad and dangerous ignorance about what is important to good health.

Questions

Because the concepts underlying both the cause and cure for TMS are unfamiliar to most people, it takes time to integrate them. Moreover, to anticipate all the questions that may arise in someone's mind is impossible. Here are some of the questions most commonly asked by patients.

Q: *"May I continue to do the exercises and stretches that I've been doing to ward off a new attack?"*

A: Many years ago I stopped prescribing physical therapy as part of the treatment program for TMS. Although the physical therapists were wonderful about emphasizing the psychological basis for the pain, each treatment session focused the patient's attention on his or her body, which was incompatible with my primary therapeutic goal of ignoring the physical and concentrating solely on the psychological. The same idea applies to any exercise routine designed to treat the back, whether it is in the form of stretching, strengthening or mobilizing.

So I advise my patients to discontinue exercises designed to protect or otherwise help the back. The back needs no protection. Warm-up exercises prior to athletic activity are appropriate for better performance but specific exercises are otherwise unnecessary.

Physical activity of all kinds is highly recommended for its psychological and general health values.

Q: *"I was in psychotherapy for over a year. Why was I still having pain if it was psychologically induced? In fact, my therapist thinks the pain is somehow psychological but she's never heard of TMS."*

A: You were still having pain because the brain would not relinquish its strategy. The pain will continue if you have not established the connection between the physical and psychologic events. Your psychotherapist, regardless of professional discipline, is not trained to make physical diagnoses and, therefore, cannot help you make that crucial link-up. You may be in psychotherapy but if you continue to take anti-inflammatory medications, undergo physical treatment for structural abnormalities and fail to acknowledge that your pain is caused by a harmless circulatory alteration induced by the brain, the pain will continue. In short, the brain will not give up the distraction unless it is forced to.

Q: *"I know I'm angry. I can feel it. In fact, I often show it. Why do I still have pain?"*

A: Because the anger you know about and express is not the anger causing your pain. TMS is a response to anger-rage generated in the unconscious (in which case you are not aware of it), or conscious anger suppressed. TMS is not a response to conscious anger felt or expressed.

   This is a subtle but important distinction. In fact, it is at the heart of the divergent approach to mindbody research. The psychologists interested in such conditions as fibromyalgia and chronic pain focus on perceived emotions like anxiety, depression and hostility. TMS theory considers these and physical disorders like TMS to be the outward manifestations of a more fundamental process that takes place in the unconscious.

   Bear in mind, we repress anger that violates our image of ourselves. For example, if I have a strong need to seek approval from everyone in my environment and someone does something that angers me, I will automatically repress that anger because it destroys my image of myself as a "nice guy." Repression is a consistent unconscious reaction that never fails. We get angry inside and do not allow it out.

   Finally, anger you are aware of may be what is known as displaced anger. That is, you become overtly angry at something relatively unimportant, like a traffic tie-up or poor service in a restaurant, instead of at your spouse or a parent, because the latter is simply not allowed by your psyche. This is very common among my patients.

Q: *"Everybody knows that I'm a calm, controlled person; that I handle everything very well and am never anxious. Why in the world should I have back pain?"*

A: Because all the personality traits that make you calm are stimulating a great deal of rage internally. The child in you says, "You're putting an enormous amount of pressure on me and that makes me furious. I want to be left alone; I want to be taken care of and you are forcing me to take care of others. I really only care about myself."

Q: *"I am the world's best coper. Why should I have back pain?"*

A: Because copers put great pressure on themselves, and the self doesn't like it at all.

Q: *"I think I know what I'm angry about inside; in fact, I'm sure it has to do with the fact that my mother constantly put me down as I was growing up. Why doesn't the pain go away?"*

A: Questions like this are common. There are three possible reasons for the persistence of symptoms. One, patients don't know *how angry* they are inside. People often find this insight very helpful and will see a reduction in pain when they realize that they are in a blind rage inside. In addition to acknowledging the anger, some people need to *feel* it directly. Then, if their symptomatology does not improve, they may want to consider psychotherapy. For some people, something other than what they think is stimulating the rage may be the culprit. They, too, will probably need to work with a psychotherapist.

Q: *"How can I tell the difference between ordinary muscle soreness and the pain of TMS?"*

A: The muscle soreness that comes on after unaccustomed physical activity tends to go away in a day or two. TMS goes on for days, weeks or months.

Location Substitution

On occasion, TMS patients will develop pain in a new location. In the lectures I describe the many variations of the syndrome, involving different muscles, nerves and tendons, so that patients will recognize a new pain when it occurs as an alternative TMS manifestation. Despite my warning that this may occur and advice to call me if it does, the tendency to attribute the new pain to something else seems irresistible.

A former patient spent a year with right foot pain that had caused substantial problems. For example, she had to work the gas and brake on her car with the left foot. When it finally occurred to her that it might be TMS, she came to see me. Once the diagnosis was established, she drove home using her right foot.

Another patient phoned me. "Cured" of her back pain about two years earlier, she'd been running regularly. Three weeks prior to her call her right hip began to hurt after a run. She saw a doctor, who diagnosed trochanteric bursitis. The prescription: a steroid injection locally and anti-inflammatory medication orally. When the pain persisted she began to think about TMS and called my office. I told her that it was a common location for TMS and that it was almost certainly a substitute for the back pain. She hung up the telephone and then, she said in a letter, "I got so angry at my brain for playing a dirty trick on me again I shouted at it, and the pain disappeared."

Often people have surgery for a substitute TMS manifestation. I had another telephone call from a woman I had treated successfully three years earlier. A few months earlier she had begun to have pain over the point of one of her shoulders. She consulted a number of shoulder experts, had an MRI that showed a torn rotator cuff, and surgery was performed to "repair the tear."

She was relieved of pain, but when she developed precisely the same pain in the opposite shoulder a few weeks later, she became suspicious and decided to call me. I told her the shoulder was a common site for TMS tendonitis and suggested an examination. At her appointment a few days later, she told me that the pain had disappeared overnight after we talked.

The rapid disappearance of new pain experienced by these patients when they learned that it was a TMS manifestation occurred because they already knew about TMS. They had gone through the period of gradual integration and assimilation of the concepts and did not have to repeat that process. As soon as they recognized the pain as part of TMS, it lost its ability to distract and promptly disappeared.

Incidentally, the almost instantaneous cessation of pain in such cases tells us something about the pathophysiology of TMS. The pain could not be the result of an inflammatory process, nor of a structural abnormality producing symptoms by compression; neither of these conditions could disappear in minutes or hours. But it is entirely compatible with a process in which the pain is due to mild oxygen deprivation, since the autonomic system can change the rate of blood flow in seconds if it so chooses.

Substitution can also occur with psychological symptoms. A young woman currently under treatment told me that she now had pain-free days but that on those days she was "an emotional basket case." Accordingly, she wanted to start psychotherapy so she could deal with the emotional turmoil "while the wound is open." I was gratified that she had learned the concepts so well. Clearly, pain and emotional states are creations of the brain for the purpose of avoidance and they can substitute for each other.

I continue to warn patients about the possibility of a location substitution, but when two or three years have passed they often forget—and experience needless discomfort.

Recurrence

Does the pain ever come back? Yes, it can—but very infrequently. Follow-up surveys have indicated that. The rate of permanent "cure" is somewhere between 90 and 95 percent.

This high "cure" rate is greatly influenced by the fact that for many years I have screened all patients before admission into the program. It would make no sense to treat people who are unable, for whatever reason, to accept the idea of a psychologically induced physical disorder. Acknowledgment and acceptance of that idea is essential to recovery.

When there is a recurrence (rarely severe), depending on circumstances, I may or may not do an examination. The patient will return for lectures or group sessions during which the reason for the return of pain is discovered and discussed. Some patients decide to start psychotherapy.

The Sine Qua Non of Treatment

I tell my patients at the end of the lectures that they must not consider themselves "cured" unless they can say unequivocally that:

> ➤ They have little or no TMS pain. A little pain of no physical or emotional consequence is permissible. We are, after all, only human.

> ➤ They are ready to engage in unrestricted physical activity.
> ➤ They have no lingering fear of any kind of physical activity.
> ➤ They have stopped all forms of physical or pharmacologic treatment.

As we learned in Part I of this book, fear is better than pain as a distractor. Therefore, unless all of these requirements are met, pain will not go away or inevitably returns. We must prove to our brains that we know what is going on, that we are not misled and, above all, that we are not intimidated or afraid. This is a contest, between our logical conscious and our irrational unconscious. It is truly a tale of two minds.

Alternative Medicine

Millions of Americans seek treatment every year from practitioners of what has been called alternative or unconventional medicine. Why? The answer is obvious. Conventional medicine has failed. This is particularly true for the musculoskeletal disorders discussed in this book. Conventional medicine has failed to cure these patients because it has failed to diagnose accurately. You cannot cure your patients if you have not identified the nature of the disease or disorder from which they suffer.

Most alternative medical treatments achieve whatever success they enjoy through the placebo effect. If the placebo phenomenon did not exist, neither would most of these treatment methods. They are potentially helpful but they do not cure because the placebo effect is almost invariably temporary.

Since most of the musculoskeletal disorders are manifestations of TMS, any treatment method that focuses on the body will perpetuate rather than halt the pain process. So, paradoxically, though the unconventional treatment may give temporary (usually partial) relief, it will often guarantee the continuation of the underlying process because it keeps the patient's attention focused on the painful body part.

I do not approve of most alternative methods of treatment for this reason. The diagnosis and treatment of TMS is not an example of unconventional or holistic medicine; it is good clinical medicine. Recognition of the causative role of emotions leads to successful diagnosis and treatment.

One alternative approach to illness is basically sound. Andrew Weil, a graduate of Harvard Medical School, a teacher and practitioner, teaches, as Norman Cousins did, that each of us has a capacity for self-healing, that we are, as Cousins says, "stronger than we think." Weil has documented the many ways we can combat disease and enhance good health beyond the methods of conventional medicine, in books like *Spontaneous Healing*.

The therapeutic approach to a pervasive medical problem described in this chapter is a specific example of the potential for self-healing that each of us possesses. It is proof that we are, indeed, stronger than we think.

A word of caution and a suggestion to readers: The many letters I have received from people who have read my books on back pain and gotten better make a strong case for the power of knowledge to reverse psychosomatic disorders. However, readers must not assume that their conditions are the result of a mindbody process unless they have been properly examined and tested by a physician and assured that they have no serious disease.

This does not mean that a psychosomatic diagnosis is made by exclusion, simply because there is no other diagnosis. However, since so few physicians make a psychosomatic diagnosis, an individual may be forced to come to that conclusion on his or her own. That is why it is essential first to rule out a nonpsychological disorder.

I receive many calls and letters from people who have decided that they have TMS and are looking for additional guidance. Unfortunately, it is both medically and ethically impossible for me to advise them. What I do suggest, if they are convinced that they have TMS or one of its equivalents, have followed their doctor's treatments and continue to have symptoms, is that they consider psychotherapy with a psychiatrist or psychologist who is trained analytically.

Closing Words

What are the most important points to remember about mindbody disorders and how to cure them?

First, that TMS and its many equivalents are essentially *harmless,* though the severity of symptoms may make that hard to believe at times.

Mindbody physical symptoms are universal in Western society; they do not imply mental or emotional illness or abnormality.

We are much *stronger* than we know, and have the capacity to influence what is going on in our bodies. But we must learn how.

Where the group of mindbody conditions described in this book is concerned, *knowledge* of the process, and most particularly knowledge of its emotional sources, is essential and almost invariably results in a "cure."

Our greatest enemies are *fear* and *misinformation.* In the realm of the emotions, we have *two minds* and must not make the mistake of judging the unconscious mind by the accepted rules of logic and rationality that are characteristic of the conscious mind.

The *mind and the body* are indivisible and in constant interaction. That makes for a magnificent organism, of infinite complexity and wonder.

Appendix: Academic Issues

This section is intended for those who are interested in the more academic aspects of mindbody medicine and, as a consequence, contains some technical terms. It should be of particular interest to psychologists and psychiatrists who follow the literature on psychosomatic medicine.

Freud and Beyond

Since TMS theory holds that the syndrome is elaborated in the unconscious to serve an unconscious purpose, it is firmly based in psychoanalytic theory. In particular, Freud's conceptualization of the unconscious provides a model for understanding the role of repression, which is of crucial importance for TMS theory. Therefore, as with so much else in the worlds of psychology and psychiatry, without Freud we would still be searching for explanations. The comparison and contrast of TMS theory with some of Freud's ideas is done with a profound sense of debt to him and his pioneering concepts.

What follows is a discussion of how TMS theory compares and contrasts with theories of psychomatosis, old and new.

Conversion Versus Psychosomatic Symptoms

Freud made a distinction between conversion hysterical symptoms and what he called the equivalents of anxiety. Early on he said that "organic" symptoms such as cardiac irregularities, diarrhea, dizziness, muscle cramps and paresthesias were not treatable by psychoanalysis, since they were not the result of hidden conflict. Instead he believed they were due to somatic sexual excitation that could not be acknowledged physically and had to seek expression by some other route, hence the affective manifestation of anxiety or a physical substitute. Later in his career he viewed anxiety as a danger signal.[1]

Experience with TMS has made it clear that psychogenic regional (conversion) and psychosomatic symptoms serve the same psychic purpose, since they can occur simultaneously in the same patient. Further, anxiety appears to be an equivalent of physical symptoms, since it often replaces them as they recede.

That the same psychology underlies both psychogenic regional and psychosomatic symptoms is reinforced by the fact that many of Freud's hysterical patients had symptoms that were clearly "vegetative." Dora had "nervous asthma" and suffered bouts of vomiting, both of which reflect altered physiology, unlike hysterical symptoms like paralysis and anesthesia, which are the result of a process elaborated entirely in the cerebrum.[2]

To my knowledge, Freud never commented on the neurophysiology of either hysterical or psychosomatic symptoms. This would be consistent with his view of himself as a psychologist, not a physiologist.

It is of interest that Freud idolized Fliess, as suggested in their early correspondence.[3] Was this partially because Fliess was preeminent as a physiologist and that then, as now, physiology and anatomy were considered the quintessential medical scientific disciplines? Early in his career Freud may have felt somewhat inferior; although he was ineluctably drawn to the creation of a new psychology, he considered it, after all, an inferior branch of science. Was his appeal to Fliess for support and encouragement based only on personal psychological need or was his loneliness and depression in part due to the fact that he was a renegade from the ranks of the "truly scientific"?

Students of psychosomatic medicine (and psychoanalysis) have always labored under feelings of inferiority, no doubt engendered by the inability to describe and define their work according to rules that govern laboratory science. If all human functions are defined in physical and chemical terms, psychosomatic medicine is not part of that science. According to that science, disease or dysfunction is the result of physical and chemical aberrations and can only be corrected by employing mechanical or chemical measures. Contemporary medicine, including much of psychiatry, seems to be governed by that philosophy.

Then how do we explain the total resolution of a painful disorder (either conversion or physiologic) through the mechanism of education, as described in this book?

Clearly, another science must be at work about which we know very little. Call it the science of the mind, or, if one adopts Bruno Bettelheim's interpretation of Freud's work, "the science of the soul or the spirit."[4] The methods of hard science cannot apply to this science. Since there is no way at present to obtain objective data pertaining to this dimension of human experience, we must rely on empirical knowledge.

Freud was justifiably confident, indeed arrogant, for he knew he had discovered something of major importance about the function of the human animal. That his theories have been modified with time is of little importance in light of their monumental contribution to human knowledge. As a true scientist he trusted his observations even though they could not be explained in physical-chemical terms.

It is now well known that mental and emotional phenomena can stimulate neuronal activity in the brain, in the process of which physical and chemical reactions are elaborated that are the progenitors of affective or physical symptoms.[5] Brain chemistry does not initiate dysfunction in this case; chemistry is in the service of the psyche. In the mindbody process the physicochemical machine is driven by the emotions, not vice versa. (The word *psyche,* derived from the Greek, means "soul.")

Physical Symptoms

Freud, as have many others, said that neurosis and symptom formation denote illness. He thought that physical symptoms had more than one meaning and represented several unconscious mental processes at the same time.[6]

The TMS model maintains that psychogenic symptom formation is universal, varying only in severity, intensity and the choice of symptom. It is the lot of all normal people and is not an illness. The psychologic purpose of physical symptoms (and of certain affective ones as well) is to divert attention from threatening rage or unbearable feelings that are the consequence of a variety of external and internal pressures.

Freud said, "The motive for being ill is, of course, invariably the gaining of some advantage." He viewed the "illness" as the means of resolving a psychic conflict; that is the primary (paranosic) gain. But he appeared to attach greater significance to the secondary (epinosic) gain derived from the "illness" as, for example, attention, sympathy and escape from responsibility or work.[7]

A fundamental disparity exists between traditional psychoanalytic theory and what has been observed in the diagnosis and treatment of TMS.

If there is an advantage to having a psychogenic symptom, as in TMS, it is the unconscious primary one of avoiding the overt expression of rage or some other unbearable feeling. Though secondary gain undoubtedly occurs (and is unconscious as well), clinical experience with TMS suggests that it is of lesser significance than primary gain.

This subject has importance that transcends a difference with traditional psychoanalytic theory, since the concept of secondary gain is currently the basis for the diagnosis and treatment of chronic pain in centers across the country. Their theory posits the existence of underlying reasons for the pain that are structural or the result of muscle deficiency disorders, and claims that the severity and chronicity of the pain are the consequence of an unconscious desire for secondary gain.[8]

In my experience with TMS, chronic pain has the same pathophysiology as acute pain; chronicity and severity are a function of the importance of the underlying psychologic state that required the pain as distraction in the first place. To base treatment on secondary gain is doubly in error: It fails to recognize the true etiology of the pain, thereby helping to perpetuate rather than ameliorate the disorder; and it misses the psychologic significance of the symptom and so cannot employ appropriate treatment. Further, it is demeaning to patients to suggest that they are deriving benefit from the malady.

Anthony Wheeler, a neurologist who sees patients at a spine center, reviewed the subject of chronic low back pain and identified contributing neurophysiologic and psychologic factors that contribute to the etiology and perpetuation of the disorder.[9] Citing many reports from the literature, he lists a variety of psychosocial phenomena such as depression, personality disorders and traits, anxiety states, substance abuse, childhood sexual abuse, anger/hostility and fear, all of which are thought to aggravate an underlying physical disorder.

In my experience psychologic factors like these contribute to or are the result of unconscious processes, which stimulate the physical symptoms characteristic of TMS that are the basis for continuing pain.

Freud concluded, "A hysterical symptom develops only where the fulfillments of two opposing wishes, arising each from a different psychical system, are able to converge in a single expression."[10]

The example he gives, not as proof but to clarify his point, is a woman with hysterical vomiting. (Vomiting is physiologic, therefore not hysterical.) Freud theorizes that one of the opposing wishes emanates from the unconscious, that she be continuously pregnant (by multiple men), and the other from the preconscious that is punishing her for that unconscious wish, since vomiting would deprive her of her figure and her good looks. He has previously stated that psychoneurotic symptoms should be regarded as fulfillments of the unconscious wishes.

TMS theory finds, by contrast, that whether the symptoms are psychosomatic or psychogenic regional (hysterical), they are designed to serve as a protective reaction to narcissistic rage or other unbearable feelings, and are not a mechanism to punish or fulfill an unconscious wish.

An alternative dynamic explanation of Freud's patient's symptoms, based on TMS theory, is that the judgmental superego is proclaiming that the woman's unconscious wishes are dangerous, preposterous, childish, even immoral, and cannot be tolerated. The narcissistic self reacts with rage to this judgment and symptoms are induced by the unconscious ego and superego as distraction, since they fear and deplore the possibility that the undesirable feeling will break out into consciousness.

In another of Freud's cases, a fourteen-year-old boy experienced "tic convulsif, hysterical vomiting, headaches, etc." when his widowed father brought home a new wife. Freud concluded that the boy was already in a suppressed rage against his father, who had upbraided him because he "played with his genitals." Though he does not say it specifically, Freud seems to be suggesting that the boy's symptoms are substituting for the rage.[11]

The interpretation from TMS theory would be that the precipitating event merely added to the boy's cumulative rage, bringing it to a critical level where it threatened to become conscious, and the onset of symptoms served to distract from the rage. Note that once again a vegetative symptom, vomiting, is identified by Freud as hysterical.

On the subject of guilt Freud said, "In the end we come to see that we are dealing with what may be called a 'moral' factor, a sense of guilt, which is finding its satisfaction in the illness and refuses to give up the punishment or suffering. We shall be right in regarding this disheartening explanation as final. But as far as the patient is concerned this sense of guilt is dumb; it does not tell him he is guilty; he does not feel guilty, he feels ill. This sense of guilt expresses itself only as a resistance to recovery which is extremely difficult to overcome."[12]

The resistance to recovery is manifest by the continuation of symptoms. Freud concluded that the repressed feeling must be guilt, since the symptom—let us call it pain—is perceived as punishment and the person must be punishing himself out of his sense of guilt. Further, Freud suggests that the feelings of inferiority "so well known in neurotics" are also a consequence of the condemnation of the ego by the hypercritical superego.

According to the TMS model, poor self-esteem is the consequence of many factors, including poor parenting, the demands of modern society, and genetic factors. The high ideals of the superego are the result of the need to demonstrate to oneself and the world that one can be perfect and good.

The TMS model holds that it is not the need to punish oneself that causes symptoms to continue but the need to divert attention from terrifying feelings that may become exposed. This is an act of *self-preservation rather than self-flagellation*. It is not a resistance to recovery, it is a resistance to *discovery*.

The superego plays a major role in repression because the coming to consciousness of feelings like rage would violate its idealistic standards of perfection. The ego participates in repression and resistance so that the whole individual will not suffer the practical consequences of rage unleased, such as condemnation, rejection and retaliation.

It has been my experience that patients whose pain resists educational therapeutic efforts are harboring repressed feelings that are deep and complicated, signaling the need for in-depth exploration, that is, psychotherapy.

What about conscious guilt? According to TMS theory only unconscious feelings produce physical symptoms. In *The Ego and Id* Freud discusses the conscious guilt in obsessional neuroses and melancholia (depression) and says it is not clear why guilt is so strong in these disorders but attributes it to the work of the superego.[13]

If one follows TMS theory, guilt is a normal consequence of demands of the superego that induce unconscious rage, which can result in physical symptoms or a variety of affective ones such as a tendency to obsess, anxiety or depression. Obsessing about symptoms is common in people with TMS, suggesting that in those patients the rage is great and the reasons for it very compelling. The basis for the choice—that is, obsession or depression—remains obscure but in either case the rage remains hidden.

As discussed in Chapter 1 of this book, depression, anxiety and obsessive-compulsive symptoms are all equivalents of TMS.

Conscious feelings, no matter how unpleasant, painful or threatening, do not cause symptoms. Only the repressed, unconscious, frightening ones necessitate either affective or physical symptoms.

Narcissistic Rage

Although Kohut fully developed the concept of narcissistic rage as the basis for affective pathology,[14] the following passage from *Beyond the Pleasure Principle* suggests that Freud had similar thoughts:

The early efflorescence of infantile sexual life is doomed to extinction because its wishes are incompatible with reality and with the inadequate state of development which the child has reached. That efflorescence comes to an end in the most distressing circumstances and to the accompaniment of the most painful feelings. Loss of love and failure leave behind them a permanent injury to self-regard in the form of a narcissistic scar, which in my opinion ... contributes more than anything to the "sense of inferiority" which is so common in neurotics.[15]

Later in the same section, Freud stated, "The lessening amount of affection he receives, the increasing demands of education, hard words and an occasional punishment—these show him at last the full extent to which he has been scorned. These are a few typical and constantly recurring instances of the ways in which the love characteristic of the age of childhood is brought to a conclusion."[16]

Here is a contribution by the master to the relevance of the idea of narcissistic rage and deep feelings of inferiority which, in my view, are universal in modern Western society, with variation in importance from person to person. They are at the heart of most psychogenic symptomatology. While Freud does not mention rage as one of the consequences of this loss of love, I doubt that he would have rejected the idea.

We would have to add, however, that not just the loss of love but a variety of other negative experiences in the developmental process contribute to injury to self-esteem and narcissistic rage.

Freud made frequent reference to deep feelings of inferiority but did not include this as a factor in the development of neuroses or symptoms. TMS theory, on the other hand, attributes perfectionism and goodism to low self-regard.

It is apparent that rage generated in infancy and childhood is permanent—put in the bank, so to speak. Deposits continue to be made to the "rage account" throughout life. Perhaps this explains why some people begin to have physical symptoms in childhood, some in their teens, others in their twenties, but the great majority in the middle years of life when the stresses and strains are the greatest. There appears to be a quantitative threshold where the level of rage, having become great enough to threaten explosion into consciousness, requires a distraction, which may be a physical symptom or an undesirable affective reaction such as anxiety, phobic or obsessive tendencies or depression.

Physical Symptoms, Anxiety, Phobia and Obsession

In discussing the significance of hysterical phobia or agoraphobia, Freud says, "Let us suppose that a neurotic patient is unable to cross the street alone—a condition which we rightly regard as a 'symptom.' If we remove this symptom by compelling him to carry out the act of which he believes himself incapable, the consequence will be an attack of anxiety; and indeed the occurrence of an anxiety attack in the street is often the precipitating cause of the onset of agoraphobia. We see, therefore, that the symptom has been constructed in order to avoid an outbreak of anxiety; the phobia is erected like a frontier fortification against anxiety."[17]

In the TMS model the symptom is erected as a distraction from rage or unbearable feelings. Both the phobia and the anxiety are "defenses," avoidance strategies in the interest of keeping the feelings unconscious. If the phobia is removed by forcing him to cross the street, the person becomes anxious. Phobias and anxiety are symptom equivalents whose purpose is to distract one's attention from repressed rage or other powerful feelings and prevent their conscious expression. It is a means of avoidance, which is a classical defense. We have said that obsessions, anxiety, depression and physical symptoms were equivalents of each other; now phobias are added to that equivalency.

The Devil and the Saint Within

Freud wrote in *The Ego and the Id*:

> One may . . . venture the hypothesis that a great part of the sense of guilt must normally remain unconscious, because the origin of conscience is intimately connected with the Oedipus complex, which belongs to the unconscious. If anyone were inclined to put forward the paradoxical proposition that the normal man is not only far more immoral than he believes but also far more moral than he knows, psychoanalysis, on whose findings the first half of the assertion rests, would have no objection to raise against the second half.[18]

Freud's assertion that the superego has its roots in the Oedipus complex stems from the idea that after passing through the stages of conflict and competition with the parent, the developing individual adopts the values of the parents and this becomes the conscience (above-I, I-ideal, superego).

It is hard to understand how these parents who have represented a variety of negative elements in the developmental process now become the personification of everything that is perfect and good, like the father-ideal, or sweet and loving, like the mother. That they have become all-perfect and all-good strains the imagination.

There seems to be more logic to the idea, "I must prove to myself and the world that I am perfect and good." The standards for these ideals are all around us: civilization, the law, religion. They are administered by parents, teachers and religious leaders. The motivation for perfection and goodness springs from deep feelings of inferiority.

TMS theory postulates that the conscience does not derive from the Oedipus complex but from multiple factors, including a deep sense of inferiority and familial, social and cultural imperatives. The dictatorial commands of the superego are designed to demonstrate both to the person himself or herself and to the world that he or she is a worthwhile (perfect), good individual. This is the saint within but there is a devil, too, in the person of that narcissistic remnant of the child that is outraged by the demands of the superego. Hence, as Freud said, at the unconscious level we are both worse and better than we know.

Whatever the roots of the superego, no one disputes its harsh, dictatorial psychic role. TMS theory says that this is enraging to the nuclear self, guided as the self is by infantile, pleasure-oriented, irresponsible wishes.

Comprehending Psychogenic Physical Symptoms

Speaking of the language of an obsessional neurosis, Freud says, "Above all, it does not involve the leap from a mental process to a somatic inner-vation—hysterical conversion—which can never be fully comprehensible to us."[19]

What Freud refers to as a leap is not so in the TMS model, which recognizes that emotions have the power to stimulate physiologic reactions of all kinds, exemplified by the symptoms in Freud's hysterical conversion patients and all of the physical processes we have designated as psychosomatic. If Freud meant that we don't know how the brain does what it does (the "black box"), then his statement applies to all mental and emotional processes, but we know enough about brain physiology to be able to link the limbic system, the hypothalamus and the autonomic and immune networks, which means that we can now explain psychogenic physical symptoms beyond the level of the "black box."[20]

The philosopher-analyst Jonathan Lear says, "Indeed, no leap is possible: not because of an unbridgeable gulf between mind and body, but because at the archaic level the body is the mind."[21]

In the adult, evidence of the archaic still exists. Although it is not the totality of the psyche it is a very important part of it. But there is powerful evidence that there is no gap and no need for a leap, in the work of Candace Pert and her colleagues who have demonstrated the information network that exists between emotional centers of the brain and the body.[22]

George McNeil described a patient with what is known as borderline personality disorder who developed a fever of unknown origin. He speculated that psychic processes could activate neuronal pathways between the limbic system and the hypothalamus leading to autonomic "disregulation," and fever.[23] This is analogous to what TMS theory says about the pain syndromes described in Part II of this book.

The Contribution of Franz Alexander

The medical literature on psychosomatic medicine has been produced almost exclusively by psychoanalysts. If TMS and its equivalents are the result of unconscious phenomena, as TMS theory holds, this is entirely appropriate, for the unconscious is the domain of the analytically trained psychotherapist. However, these workers are at a disadvantage in their study of the problem since they do not have awareness of and access to the full range of people with mindbody disorders. As a result, their theories on the nature of psychogenesis may lack precision.

Frosch[24] pointed out the fact that Franz Alexander, founder of the Chicago Institute for Psychoanalysis, and his colleagues French and Pollock made a major contribution to the field of psychosomatic medicine in the twentieth century and came close to achieving acceptance of its concepts by mainstream medicine.[25] Alas, it was not to be.

Alexander included a large number of maladies in his definition of *psychosomatic* but neither he nor his successors were aware of the most common psychosomatic manifestations, the neuromusculoskeletal maladies that are the main subject of this book.

Alexander introduced the concept of "vegetative neuroses," referring to what have been designated psychosomatic, as opposed to conversion disorders, in his book. In Alexander's classification, these included migraine, hypertension, hyperthyroidism, cardiac neuroses, rheumatoid arthritis, vasopressor syncope, peptic ulcer, ulcerative colitis, constipation, diarrhea, fatigue states, and asthma.

He related specific unconscious conflicts to specific physical disorders but did not make the distinction between conversion and psychosomatic symptoms suggested in Chapter 2 of this book. Alexander noted, as

I have, that Freud often referred to symptoms that were clearly psychosomatic as though they were conversion—therefore, the result of unconscious conflict.

TMS theory is in complete accord with this view, though it differs in the nature of the unconscious process responsible for symptoms, in the purpose of symptoms and in the principle of specificity. Despite the difference in detail, there is continuity and support for TMS theory in the work of Freud and Alexander. The concept of overriding importance is that symptoms are the result of unconscious phenomena, although that idea is repudiated by some contemporary theorists.[26]

It is interesting to compare and contrast the major tenets of Alexander's theories with TMS theory:

1. Alexander believed personality qualities derived early in life play a major role in the evolution of psychosomatic symptoms. TMS theory is in complete agreement, especially if those qualities include the need to be perfect and good.
2. Alexander believed stressful life events or circumstances activate emotional processes in the unconscious, resulting in symptoms. Agreed. These events generate internal rage, since they represent pressure on the narcissistic self.
3. Alexander's group attributed choice of organ and symptom to a constitutionally determined factor they called "X."

Based on empirical evidence derived from clinical experience with many thousands of patients, TMS theory finds that the same psychologic stimulus results in symptoms that may move from one organ or system to another, and no evidence of genetic, biochemical or physiologic determinants. It postulates different levels of physiologic involvement, with TMS and its equivalents representing the least serious, and the autoimmune, cardiovascular and cancer categories the more severe. Though it is likely that emotions play a role in the etiology of the more serious disorders, *what that role is has yet to be determined.*

Why the brain chooses the parts of the body and symptoms that it does is a subject of great interest. One can only speculate on that process within the category of TMS and its equivalents.

Edward Shorter, a medical historian, has written persuasively on this subject and has concluded that people unconsciously choose a disorder that is *in vogue* and is considered *a legitimate physical disorder* by the medical community.[27] One might call this "social contagion." I agree with this explanation for symptom choice.

Two striking examples are disorders that are responsible for a high proportion of disability due to pain in the United States:

1. The whole range of low back, neck, shoulder and limb pain syndromes—TMS.
2. The syndromes of repetitive stress injuries (RSI). They are also part of TMS.

These two groups affect an enormous number of people but *are never diagnosed as psychosomatic.* Patients prefer a nonpsychologic, structural diagnosis, and practitioners from a variety of disciplines are ready to oblige them. The setting is perfect for an epidemic.

If a symptom is successfully treated, as peptic ulcer can be through the use of potent pharmacologic agents, the psyche simply looks elsewhere. This is a common observation and in most cases the alternative location remains within category. For example, the site may move from stomach to back pain, or neck pain to headache. New locations within the TMS syndrome itself are frequent: for example, from back to neck to knee or shoulder.

I theorize that the choice of category—that is, TMS and its equivalents or an autoimmune disease, one of the serious cardiovascular conditions or cancer—may be a function of the severity and intensity of the emotional state. It is possible that more severe emotional states are more deeply repressed and that may be a factor in disease choice.

Finally, I have had many patients who have moved from more severe psychosomatic manifestations to milder ones: bulimia or anorexia nervosa to back pain, for example. My interpretation is that they have improved psychologically and no longer require the more powerful distraction. Once more, the intensity of the psychologic state is a factor in symptom choice.

Alexander went beyond Freud in suggesting that the vegetative symptoms were the result of conflictual processes and were, therefore, amenable to analytically oriented therapy.

TMS theory and practice agrees with Alexander and has demonstrated that such symptoms are treatable. It holds that the major conflict is between the tyrannical, despotic superego and the protesting, narcissistic self.

Heinz Kohut

Going conceptually and historically beyond Freud and Alexander, theories of psychogenesis and psychosomatosis based on experience with TMS also depend for their structure on the Self Psychology concepts of Heinz Kohut, a noted analyst who published in the seventies and eighties.[28]

From the beginning it was apparent that certain personality traits play an important role in the genesis of psychosomatic disorders; they are the superego-inspired compulsions to be perfect and/or good. The question was, What is the link between these traits and physical symptoms? Kohut's theory of narcissistic rage filled the gap.

Kohut originated the body of theory now known as Self Psychology. Fundamental to his theory is the idea that there is a developmental process in infancy in which the child derives responses from its mother (who is known as the selfobject in Self Psychology parlance) that are essential for its normal emotional growth and development. Under optimal circumstances the self in the child has experiences of being admired, affirmed, praised and valued, called mirroring of the grandiose self. Calming, soothing experiences that come from its feeling of having merged with the powerful parental figure coupled with reassuring strengthening feelings of alikeness with the mother, called twinship, further contribute to the development of a healthy self.

Kohut held that psychopathology was based on "defects in the structure of the self, on distortions of the self, or on weakness of the self," and that these were the result of a mismatch between mother and child. The mother's contribution to the mismatch is obvious if she has psychological problems but may also come from cultural or societal imperatives. Presumably, the infant's contribution is based on genetic factors.

The child whose psychological needs are not adequately met becomes the adult with problems, among them what are known as narcissistic personality disorders, characterized by narcissistic rage.

This theory represents a distinct departure from the classical drive model of psychopathology in suggesting that the rage results from self deficits. Therefore, according to Kohut, therapy must be designed to heal the narcissistic wounds, so to speak, rather than confronting the patient with what is going on in the unconscious; healing rather than revealing the conflict.

How does this play out in the adult and, particularly, how does it relate to TMS?

Kohut theorized that there is a separate developmental line for narcissism that, adequately nurtured through infancy and the ensuing stages of life, leads to an adult self that is normally narcissistic, mature, cohesive and healthy. The pathological state exists when the deficient self is easily injured and, therefore, in a state of perpetual rage. Self Psychology theory states that rage is a "disintegration product" following narcissistic injury and that symptoms are a physical expression of rage.

TMS theory sees rage as a normal reaction of the residual child in each of us to narcissistic injury. Intellectually, we are strongly impelled to find a logical excuse for the rage, since we find it hard to acknowledge such a primitive, excessive reaction to the injury. We must accept the rage as normal for the residual child in us.

TMS theory needed the concept of narcissistic rage to fully explain mindbody disorders. But the TMS model of psychosomatosis goes further, suggesting that narcissism and narcissistic rage are universal. This is based on the observation that psychosomatic symptoms are universal among normal people, of all ages and both sexes. So we reason backward, from the soma to the psyche. If psychosomatic symptoms exist for the purpose of diverting attention from unconscious rage, and everyone has psychosomatic symptoms, then everyone must have some unconscious rage. This we believe to be true and suggest that the lack of knowledge of this basic fact helps to account for the pain epidemic and a variety of other disorders in Western society.

Stanley Coen

I am indebted to Columbia psychoanalyst Stanley Coen for his suggestion that the symptoms of TMS are not anxiety equivalents but manifestations of an avoidance process. This idea was of crucial importance in conceptualizing TMS, for at one fell swoop it identified the purpose of physical symptomatology, on the one hand, and the reason why patients were "cured" by cognitive-analytic therapy, on the other. The physical symptoms were distracting the patients, diverting their attention from the psychic to the physical, assisting the process of repression in its important task of preventing exteriorization of the dreaded rage. My program was blowing the cover on this covert operation, rendering it null and void. With awareness of the existence of unconscious rage, patients no longer need a distraction, which leads nicely into the next question.

Can the Unconscious Become Conscious?

This is an issue of some importance; it bears on the physiology of psychosomatic disorders as well as questions of therapeutic strategy.

Graeme Taylor

In his book *Psychosomatic Medicine and Contemporary Psychoanalysis,* Graeme Taylor, a Canadian psychoanalyst, says, "there are clinical indications, too, that dreams are not instigated solely by the unconscious mind. If they were, then as psychoanalysis or psychoanalytic psychotherapy *rendered the unconscious conscious* [my italics], one would expect a reduction in the number of dreams. But insight does not result in fewer dreams."[29]

There is an important misconception here. Insight does not render the unconscious conscious; it merely makes one aware of the existence of repressed emotions. In many years of diagnosing and treating a psychosomatic disorder induced by repressed rage, I know of only one person whose feelings broke through into consciousness (see pages 12–15). Psychotherapists who work with me report that they only see this process occasionally. But that does not mean we no longer generate and repress feelings. Powerful but frightening feelings recur constantly and they continue to accumulate and be repressed.

Of course insight does not result in fewer dreams, because insight does not render the unconscious conscious. The process of repression is extremely efficient, which is why affective and psychosomatic symptoms are universal. They signify the triumph of repression.

This does not imply that repressed emotions are not trying to come to consciousness. This is at the heart of the psychosomatic process. This drive to consciousness, the threat that what is repressed will become overt, consciously felt and expressed, creates the need for a distraction, hence a physical or affective symptom.

Lear has described this drive as "a yearning for expression" or a "unification of thought and feeling."[30] He does so in the context of whether what Freud and Breuer called catharsis was really that or rather the attempt to unify thought and feeling, which Lear considered to be very different psychodynamically. He says that it was not discharge of feelings but their recognition that effected the cure. This is precisely what we have observed in the majority of successfully treated patients with TMS.

For most TMS patients, merely making them aware that their symptoms are psychologically induced and listing the major psychologic factors at work is enough to stop symptoms. They do not have a "cathartic experience"—they acquire knowledge. As noted earlier, the conscious experience of strongly repressed feelings is relatively rare. Analytically oriented psychotherapy over long periods of time may bring patients to experience previously repressed emotions, but there may be multiple ranks of defense to prevent that from happening.

Neurobiology, Psychobiology and Disregulation

This is not the place for a thorough discussion of alternative theories of psychosomatosis. However, it is desirable to touch on one of them, since it bears on the validity of TMS theory.

Taylor expresses the theoretical basis for TMS succinctly: "The traditional psychosomatic model of disease is one in which stressful environmental events and/or intrapsychic conflicts evoke certain states of mind which lead to altered physiology and eventually to pathological changes in bodily function and structure. This linear model assumes that the psychological and physiological responses to life experiences are casually related and involve the same neural processes."[31] He then goes on to reject this model in favor of a new one.

TMS follows the linear model. It does not need a new one. Our consistent therapeutic success, based primarily on awareness and possibly some degree of empathic concern, parallels Freud's success with his hysterical patients. We see no need for alternative theories.

The heart of the new model appears to be the idea that psychosocial phenomena and external stimuli can alter the body directly and need not do so exclusively by their impact on the mind. From this basic idea an elaborate structure has been hypothesized using general systems theory, biofeedback, self-regulation and disregulation concepts to explain what happens in health and illness.

Taylor cites as an example[32] a study reporting that the longevity of male survivors of myocardial infarction was significantly greater in those who enjoyed good social relationships than in their socially isolated counterparts.

One fails to see, however, how this supports the new model. To be sure the old model has not yet worked out all the details of how either positive or negative life experiences affect body function, but neither has the new one. The TMS experience provides a clear description of how one category of psychosomatic disorders occurs, and it does not need the concepts of psychobiological disregulation to explain it.

The new theories suggest that dual processes are at work; that psychologically supportive phenomena can work on the mind and body simultaneously, or conversely, people who were psychologically deprived during childhood will have certain psychic defects as adults but will also be "disregulated" physically. This is how they conclude that psychosomatic manifestations are the result of a direct effect on target organs rather than through the brain.

If this were so, there would be no way to explain the therapeutic results of TMS therapy, for the disappearance of symptoms is mediated directly through the brain. The person becomes aware—the pain ceases.

A case history of one of Taylor's own patients was most instructive. She was a forty-two-year-old divorced woman who presented a variety of psychosomatic symptoms. She was self-supporting, enmeshed in a demanding relationship with an elderly mother and had few social supports. Taylor initiated behavioral treatment but did tell her that the original symptoms were related to the situation with her mother. He described himself as a selfobject who was performing a regulatory function. When he tried to terminate the therapeutic relationship the patient developed Bell's palsy.

My interpretation of this case is that the patient was enraged by her entrapment by her mother, lack of a partner (divorced), and social supports. Taylor must be a personable doctor, and he soothed her rage over her social and personal problems by consenting to treat her. He chose muscle relaxation techniques but provided insight by telling her that her symptoms were related to inner conflict about the relationship with her mother. It may not have made any difference what therapeutic method he chose because this supportive doctor was caring for her, soothing her rage, in fact, probably providing her with all of Kohut's empathic supports—and so her original symptoms abated.

Then he abandoned her! That was the crowning blow. Now her rage increased to a "dangerous" level, that is, to the point where it threatened to escape repression and become conscious. Of all things (her unconscious tells her), it would be unpardonable to be enraged at this good doctor who had helped her. So the psyche did what it must to distract her—it created a mononeuropathy of the right seventh cranial nerve, almost certainly through the psychosomatic mechanism that characterizes

TMS, that is, autonomically mediated local ischemia. Bell's palsy is one of the mononeuropathies I list as possible neural manifestations of TMS.

Taylor's case is an excellent example of how the TMS process works. It also suggests that there is no need to talk of a "regulatory function," though one should retain Kohut's selfobject designation. He was not regulating her; he was informing and caring for her.

To summarize the psychodynamic events in Taylor's case, a concatenation of personality traits and life circumstances had created sufficient narcissistic rage to mandate the creation of physical symptoms, those the patient had when she first consulted Taylor. He treated her, the symptoms abated, and then he abandoned her.

The case confirms the therapeutic value of helping patients identify the sources of rage, a fundamental principle in the treatment of TMS. Taylor informed the patient that "conflict" in the relationship with her mother was responsible for her symptoms (all of which were classic for TMS, incidentally). He also administered a liberal dose of Kohut's empathy, which in this case may have been the more important therapeutic ingredient. In my clinical experience insight seems to be primary, which is particularly well illustrated in those patients who have been "cured" by reading one of my books.

It would appear that the need for the new model of psychosomatic disease suggested by Taylor reflects the failure of contemporary medicine to explain and successfully treat psychosomatic disorders, on the one hand, and a compulsion to join the ranks of the "scientific" on the other. As psychoanalysis began to fall out of favor with psychiatrists, it was no longer acceptable as the theoretical basis for psychosomatosis and so a new theory was required. And, of course, it would have to be one that would be acceptable to "hard science"; hence the concepts of "structural psychic defects" or the neuroanatomical defects postulated for people who are diagnosed with alexithymia.

That term has been applied to patients who do not verbally express their feelings and appear not even to recognize them. Nemiah, a student of psychosomatic medicine, has proposed that this is a separate, distinct disorder and, as noted earlier, may be related to structural brain defects.[33]

I am in agreement with McDougall, who believes the observed behavior of alexithymic patients represents a defense against frightening feelings.[34] The behavior is frequently seen in TMS patients who are referred for psychotherapy. All of them have symptoms of physical pain, so they are classically psychosomatic and are not aware, as McDougall suggested, that their problems are psychic in origin. That signals massive denial by the patient, a state that does not justify the creation of another psychologic diagnosis. Lesser and Lesser have warned against imbuing a theoretical concept like alexithymia with a material existence.[35]

One cannot help but reflect that pure, "linear" psychosomatic concepts have never had a chance to develop. Alexander started the process but no one continued his work.

Laboring under the inferiority complex noted earlier, and because they have had to account for their views on empirical rather than laboratory grounds, many psychoanalysts have eagerly accepted theories that sound more "scientific." The theory of psychosomatosis put forth in this book does not require cybernetically derived concepts to explain its diagnostic or therapeutic rationales. Further, it has been put to the test successfully, so it must be accurate.

The realm of the emotions and emotionally induced symptomatology remains shrouded in mystery and will probably remain so until we know how the brain functions at a very basic level. Neither physics, chemistry nor cybernetics will unravel that mystery. The solution may require a new epistemology. Until then we must be content to make careful observations and have the scientific integrity to act upon them responsibly.

Notes

1. S. Freud, *Complete Psychological Works* (London: Hogarth Press, 1953–1961), XX: 87–174.

2. Ibid., VII: 7–63.

3. S. J. Coen, *Between Author and Reader* (New York: Columbia University Press, 1994).

4. B. Bettelheim, "Freud and the Soul," in *The New Yorker,* March 1, 1982.

5. C. B. Pert, *Molecules of Emotion* (New York: Scribner's, 1997); S. Reichlin, "Neuroendocrine-immune interactions," in *New England Journal of Medicine* 329 (1993): 1246–1253.

6. Freud, *Works,* VII: 47.

7. Ibid., VII: 43.

8. W. E. Fordyce, *Behavioral Methods for Chronic Pain and Illness* (St. Louis: C. V. Mosby, 1976).

9. A. H. Wheeler, "Evolutionary Mechanisms in Chronic Low Back Pain and Rationale for Treatment," in *American Journal of Pain Management* 5 (1995): 62–66.

10. Freud, *Works,* V: 569.

11. Ibid., V: 619.

12. Ibid., XIX: 48–59.

13. Ibid.

14. H. Kohut, *The Analysis of the Self* (New York: International Universities Press, 1971).

15. Freud, *Works* XVIII: 20.

16. Ibid., XVIII: 21.

17. Ibid., V: 581–582.

18. Ibid., XIX: 48–59.

19. Ibid., X.

20. Pert, *Molecules of Emotion;* Reichlin, "Neuroendocrine-immune Interactions."

21. J. Lear, *Love and Its Place in Nature: A Philosophical Interpretation of Freudian Psychoanalysis* (New York: Farrar, Strauss and Giroux, 1990), 39.

22. Pert, *Molecules of Emotion.*

23. G. N. McNeil, L. H. Leighton, and A. M. Elkins, "Possible Psychogenic Fever of 103 F in a Patient with Borderline Personality Disorder," in *American Journal of Psychiatry* 141 (1984): 896–897.

24. J. Frosch, *Psychodynamic Psychiatry* (Madison, Conn.: International Universities Press, 1990).

25. F. Alexander, *Psychosomatic Medicine* (New York: W. W. Norton, 1950); F. Alexander, T. M. French and G. H. Pollock, *Psychosomatic Specificity* (University of Chicago Press, 1968).

26. Z. J. Lipowski, "Somatization: The Concept and Its Clinical Application," in *American Journal of Psychiatry* 145 (1988): 1358–1368; M. F. Reiser, *Mind, Brain, Body* (New York: Basic Books, 1984); E. L. Rossi, *The Psychobiology of Mind-Body Healing* (New York: W. W. Norton, 1986).

27. E. Shorter, *From Paralysis to Fatigue: A History of Psychosomatic Illness in the Modern Era* (New York: The Free Press, 1992).

28. Kohut, *Analysis of the Self;* H. Kohut and E. Wolf, "The Disorders of the Self and Their Treatment," in *International Journal of Psychoanalysis* 59 (1978): 413–425.

29. G. J. Taylor, *Psychosomatic Medicine and Contemporary Psychoanalysis* (Madison, Conn.: International Universities Press, 1987), 203.

30. Lear, *Love and Its Place.*

31. Taylor, *Psychosomatic Medicine,* 279.

32. Ibid., 287.

33. J. C. Nemiah, "Alexithymia: Theoretical Considerations," in *Psychotherapy and Psychosomatics* 28 (1977): 199–206.

34. J. McDougall, *Theaters of the Body* (New York: W. W. Norton, 1989).

35. I. M. Lesser and B. Z. Lesser, "Alexithymia: Examining the Development of a Psychological Concept," in *American Journal of Psychiatry* 140 (1983): 1305–1308.

Bibliography

Abbey, S. E., and Garfinkel, P. E. "Neurasthenia and chronic fatigue syndrome: the role of culture in the making of a diagnosis." *American Journal of Psychiatry* 148 (1991): 1638–1641.

Alexander, F. *Psychosomatic Medicine*. New York: W. W. Norton, 1950.

Alexander, F., French, T. M., and Pollock, G. H. *Psychosomatic Specificity*. Chicago: University of Chicago Press, 1968.

Beecher, H. K. "Pain in men wounded in battle." *Annals of Surgery* 123 (1946): 96–105.

Bengtsson, A., and Bengtsson, M. "Regional sympathetic blockade in primary fibromyalgia." *Pain* 33 (1988): 161–167.

Benson, H. *Timeless Healing*. New York: Scribner, 1996.

Bettelheim, B., "Freud and the soul." *The New Yorker,* March 1, 1982.

Bigos S. J., et al. "A prospective study of work perceptions and psychosocial factors affecting the report of back injury." *Spine* 16 (1991): 1–6.

Blumer, D., and Heilbronn, M. "Chronic pain as a variant of depressive illness." *Journal of Nervous and Mental Disease* 170 (1982): 381–406.

Bowen, C. D. *The Most Dangerous Man in America*. Boston: Little, Brown, 1974.

Bozzao, A., et al. "Lumbar disk herniation: MR imaging assessment of natural history in patients treated without surgery." *Radiology* 185 (1992): 135–141.

Cannito, M. P. "Emotional considerations in spasmodic dysphonia: psychometric quantification." *Journal of Communicative Disorders* 24 (1991): 313–329.

Chopra, D. *Quantum Healing*. New York: Bantam Books, 1989.

Coen, S. J. *Between Author and Reader*. New York: Columbia University Press, 1994.

Cousins, N. *Anatomy of an Illness*. New York: W. W. Norton, 1979.

Deyo, R. A. "Fads in the treatment of low back pain." *New England Journal of Medicine.* 325 (1991): 1039–1040.

Deyo, R. A., Loeser, J. D., and Bigos, S. T. "Herniated lumbar intervertebral disk." *Annals of Internal Medicine* 112 (1990): 598–603.

Deyo, R. A. "Practice variations, treatment fads, rising disability." *Spine* 18 (1993): 2153–2162.

Diagnostic and Statistical Manual of Mental Disorders, Fourth Edition. Washington, DC: American Psychiatric Association, 1994.

Duffy, J. R. *Motor Speech Disorders.* St. Louis: Mosby Year Book, 1995.

Edelman, G. M. *Bright Air, Brilliant Fire.* New York: Basic Books, 1992.

Eisenberg, D. M., et al. "Unconventional medicine in the United States." *New England Journal of Medicine* 328 (1993): 246–252.

Epstein, A. *Mind, Fantasy and Healing.* New York: Delacorte Press, 1994.

Esterling, B. A., et al. "Emotional disclosure through writing or speaking modulates latent Epstein-Barr virus antibody titers." *Journal of Consulting and Clinical Psychology* 62 (1994): 130–140.

Fassbender, H. G., and Wegner, K. "Morphologie and pathogenese des weichteilrheumatismus." *Z. Rheumaforsch* 32 (1973): 355–360.

Fassbender, H. G. *Pathology of Rheumatic Diseases.* New York: Springer, 1985.

Fernandez, E., and Turk, D. C. "The scope and significance of anger in the experience of chronic pain." *Pain* 61 (1995): 165–175.

Flor, H., Turk, D. C., and Birbaumer, N. "Assessment of stress related psychophysiological reactions in chronic back pain patients." *Journal of Consulting and Clinical Psychology* 53 (1985): 354–364.

Fordyce, W. E. *Behavioral Methods for Chronic Pain and Illness.* St. Louis: C. V. Mosby, 1976.

Fox, A. J., et al. "Myelographic cervical nerve root deformities." *Radiology* 116 (1975): 355–361.

Freud, Sigmund. *The Complete Psychological Works of Sigmund Freud.* Standard Edition. 24 vols. London: Hogarth Press, 1953–1961.

Friedman, M., and Rosenman, R. *Type A Behavior and Your Heart.* New York: Knopf, 1984.

Frieman, B. G., Albert, T. J., and Fenlin, J. M. "Rotator cuff disease: a review of diagnosis, pathophysiology, and current trends in treatment." *Archives of Physical Medicine and Rehabilitation* 75 (1994): 604–609.

Frosch, J. *Psychodynamic Psychiatry.* Madison, CT: International Universities Press, 1990.

Gay, P. *Freud: A Life for Our Time.* New York: W. W. Norton, 1988.

Gaylin, W. *The Rage Within.* New York: Simon & Schuster, 1984.

Goldenberg, D. L. "Fibromyalgia, chronic fatigue syndrome, and myofascial pain syndrome." *Current Opinion in Rheumatology* 5 (1993): 199–208.

Gore, R. D., Sepic, M.S., and Gardner, G. M. "Roentgenographic findings of the cervical spine in asymptomatic people." *Spine* 11 (1986): 521–524.

Gould, S. J. "This view of life." *Natural History,* June 1986.

Gould, S. J. "This view of life." *Natural History,* January 1991.

Grady, D. "In one country, chronic whiplash is uncompensated (and unknown)." *New York Times,* May 7, 1996 (Section C3).

Haldane, J. B. S. *Possible Worlds and Other Essays.* London: Chatto & Windus, 1927.

Heilbroner, D. "Repetitive stress injury." *Working Woman,* February 1993, pp. 61–65.

Henriksson, K. G., and Bengtsson, A. "Fibromyalgia: a clinical entity?" *Canadian Journal of Physiological Pharmacology* 69 (1991): 672–677.

Holmes, T. H., and Rahe, R. H. "The Social Readjustment Rating Scale." *Journal of Psychosomatic Research* 11 (1967): 213–218.

Jensen, M. C., et al. "Magnetic resonance imaging of the lumbar spine in people without back pain." *New England Journal of Medicine* 331 (1994): 69–73.

Klein, L. M., Lavker, R. M., Matis, W. L., and Murphy, G. E. "Degranulation of human mast cells induces an endothelial antigen central to leukocyte adhesion." *Proceedings of the National Academy of Sciences* 86 (1989): 8972–8976.

Kohut, H. *The Analysis of the Self.* New York: International Universities Press, 1971.

Kohut, H., and Wolf, E. "The disorders of the self and their treatment." *International Journal of Psychoanalysis* 59 (1978): 413–425.

Lalli, A. F. "Urographic contrast media reactions and anxiety." *Radiology* 112 (1974): 267–271.

Larsson, S. E., et al. "Chronic pain after soft tissue injury of the cervical spine: trapezius muscle blood flow and electromyography at static loads and fatigue." *Pain* 57 (1994): 173–180.

Lear, J. *Love and Its Place in Nature: A Philosophical Interpretation of Freudian Psychoanalysis.* New York: Farrar, Strauss and Giroux, 1990.

LeShan, L. *You Can Fight For Your Life.* New York: Evans, 1977.

Lesser, I. M., and Lesser, B. Z. "Alexithymia: Examining the development of a psychological concept." *American Journal of Psychiatry* 140 (1983): 1305–1308.

Lipowski, Z. J. "Somatization: the concept and its clinical application." *American Journal of Psychiatry* 145 (1988): 1358–1368.

Locke, S., and Colligan, D. *The Healer Within.* New York: E. P. Dutton, 1986.

Ludlow, C. L., and Connor, N. P. "Dynamic aspects of phonatory control in spasmodic dysphonia." *Journal of Speech and Hearing Research* 30 (1987): 197–206.

Lund, N., Bengtsson, A., and Thorborg, P. "Muscle tissue oxygen pressure in primary fibromyalgia." *Scandinavian Journal of Rheumatology* 15 (1986): 165–173.

Magora, A., and Schwartz, A. "Relation between the low back pain syndrome and x-ray findings 1. Degenerative osteoarthritis." *Scandinavian Journal of Rehabilitation Medicine* 8 (1976): 115–125.

Magora, A., and Schwartz, A. "Relation between the low back pain syndrome and x-ray findings 2. Transitional vertebra (mainly sacralization)." *Scandinavian Journal of Rehabilitation Medicine* 10 (1978): 135–145.

Magora, A., and Schwartz, A. "Relation between the low back pain syndrome and x-ray findings 3. Spina bifida occulta." *Scandinavian Journal of Rehabilitation Medicine* 12 (1980): 9–15.

Malmivaara, A., et al. "The treatment of acute low back pain—bed rest, exercise or ordinary activity?" *New England Journal of Medicine* 332 (1995): 351–355.

Mann, S. J. "Stress and hypertension—the role of unintegrated emotions: revival of a hypothesis." *Integrative Psychiatry* 8 (1992): 191–197.

Mann, S. J., and Delon, M. "Improved hypertension control after disclosure of decades-old trauma." *Psychosomatic Medicine* 57 (1995): 501–505.

Mann, S. J. "Severe paroxysmal hypertension: an automatic syndrome and its relationship to repressed emotions." *Psychosomatics* 37 (1996): 444–450.

McCain, G. A. "Fibromyalgia and myofascial pain syndromes." In Wall, P. D., and Melzack, R., *Textbook of Pain* (3rd edition). Edinburgh and New York: Churchill Livingstone, 1994.

McDougall, J. *Theaters of the Body.* New York: Norton, 1989.

McNeil, G. N. Leighton, L. H., and Elkins, A. M. "Possible psychogenic fever of 103°F in a patient with borderline personality disorder." *American Journal of Psychiatry* 141 (1984): 896–897.

McRae, D. L. "Asymptomatic intervertebral disc protrusions." *Acta Radiologica* 46 (1965): 9–27.

Miller, H. C. "Stress prostatitis." *Urology* 32 (1988): 507–510.

Mixter, W. J., and Barr, J. S. "Rupture of the intervertebral disc with involvement of the spinal cord." *New England Journal of Medicine* 211 (1934): 210–214.

Mountz, J. M., et al. "Fibromyalgia in women." *Arthritis & Rheumatism* 38 (1995): 926–938.

Nachemson, A. L. "The lumbar spine: an orthopedic challenge." *Spine* 1 (1976): 59–71.

Nemiah, J. C. "Alexithymia: theoretical considerations." *Psychotherapy and Psychosomatics* 28 (1977): 199–206.

Ornish, D., et al. "Can lifestyle changes reverse coronary heart disease?" *The Lancet* 336 (1990): 129–133.

Pellegrino, M. J., et al. "Prevalence of mitral valve prolapse in primary fibromyalgia: a pilot investigation." *Archives of Physical Medicine and Rehabilitation* 70 (1989): 541–543.

Pelletier, K. R. *Mind as Healer, Mind as Slayer.* New York: Dell, 1977.

Pennebaker, J. W., Kiecolt-Glaser, J., and Glaser, R. "Disclosure of traumas and immune function: health implications for psychotherapy." *Journal of Consulting and Clinical Psychology* 56 (1988): 239–245.

Pert, C. B. *Molecules of Emotion.* New York: Scribner, 1997.

Quint, M. "Bane of insurers: new ailments." *New York Times,* Nov. 28, 1994 (Section D1).

Reichlin, S. "Neuroendocrine-immune interactions." *New England Journal of Medicine* 329 (1993): 1246–1253.

Reiser, M. F. *Mind, Brain, Body.* New York: Basic Books, 1984.

Rosomoff, H. L. *Do Herniated Discs Produce Pain? Advances in Pain Research and Therapy* (Vol. 9), edited by H. L. Fields et al. New York: Raven Press, 1985.

Rosomoff, H. L., and Rosomoff, R. S. "Nonsurgical aggressive treatment of lumbar spinal stenosis." *Spine* 1 (1987): 383–400.

Rossi, E. L. *The Psychobiology of Mind-Body Healing.* New York: Norton, 1986.

Saal, J. S., Saal, J. A., and Yurth, E. F. "Nonoperative management of herniated cervical intervertebral disc with radiculopathy." *Spine* 21 (1996): 1877–1883.

Sarno, J. E. "Psychogenic backache: the missing dimension." *Journal of Family Practice* 1 (1974): 8–12.

Sarno, J. E. "Chronic back pain and psychic conflict." *Scandinavian Journal of Rehabilitation Medicine* 8 (1976): 143–153.

Sarno, J. E. "Psychosomatic backache." *Journal of Family Practice* 5 (1974): 353–357.

Sarno, J. E. "Etiology of neck and back pain: an autonomic myoneuralgia?" *Journal of Nervous and Mental Disease* 69 (1981): 55–59.

Sarno, J. E. "Therapeutic Exercise for Back Pain." In *Therapeutic Exercise* (4th edition), J. V. Basmajian, ed. Baltimore: Williams and Wilkins, 1984.

Sarno, J. E. *Mind Over Back Pain.* New York: William Morrow, 1984.

Sarno, J. E. "Psychosomatic back pain alias lumbar herniated disc pain." Unpublished manuscript.

Sarno, J. E. *Healing Back Pain.* New York: Warner Books, 1991.

Schnall, P. L., et al. "The relationship between 'job strain,' workplace diastolic blood pressure, and left ventricular mass." *Journal of the American Medical Association* 263 (1990): 1929–1935.

Schrader, H., et al. "Natural evolution of late whiplash syndrome outside the medicolegal context." *Lancet* 347 (1996): 1207–1211.

Schwaber, E. "On the 'self' within the matrix of analytic theory: some clinical reflections and reconsiderations." *International Journal of Psychoanalysis* 60 (1979): 467–479.

Schwartz, J. M., et al. "Systematic change in cerebral glucose metabolic rate after successful behavior modification treatment of obsessive-compulsive disorder." *Archives of General Psychiatry* 53 (1996): 109–113.

Shorter, E. *From Paralysis to Fatigue: A History of Psychosomatic Illness in the Modern Era.* New York and Toronto: The Free Press, 1992.

Siegel, B. S. *Love, Medicine and Miracles.* New York: Harper & Row, 1986.

Simonton, O. C., Matthews-Simonton, S., and Creighton, J. L. *Getting Well Again.* New York: Bantam Books, 1981.

Smedslund, J. "How shall the concept of anger be defined?" *Theoretical Psychology* 3 (1992): 5–34.

Smyth, J. M., et al. "Effects of writing about stressful experiences on symptom reduction in patients with asthma or rheumatoid arthritis." *Journal of the American Medical Association* 281 (1999): 1304–1309.

Sorotzkin, B. "The quest for perfection: avoiding guilt or avoiding shame?" *Psychotherapy* 22 (1985): 564–570.

Spiegel, W. "Emotional expression and disease outcome." *Journal of the American Medical Association* 281 (1999): 1328–1329.

Sunderland, S. *Nerve Injuries and Their Repair: A Critical Appraisal.* Edinburgh: Churchill Livingstone, 1991.

Swanson, D. W. "Chronic pain as a third pathologic emotion." *American Journal of Psychiatry* 141 (1984): 210–214.

Taylor, G. J. *Psychosomatic Medicine and Contemporary Psychoanalysis* Madison, CT: International Universities Press, 1987.

Thompson, J. M. "Tension myalgia as a diagnosis at the Mayo Clinic and its relationship to fibrositis, fibromyalgia, and myofascial pain syndrome." *Mayo Clinic Proceedings* 65 (1990): 1237–1248.

Turner, J. A., et al. "The importance of placebo effects in pain treatment and research." *Journal of the American Medical Association* 271 (1994): 1609–1614.

Unsigned editorial. "Autonomic function in mitral valve prolapse." *The Lancet,* Oct. 3, 1987: 773–774.

Walters, A. "Psychogenic regional pain alias hysterical pain." *Brain* 84 (1961): 1–18.

Weil, A. *Spontaneous Healing.* New York: Knopf, 1995.

Wheeler, A. H. "Evolutionary mechanisms in chronic low back pain and rationale for treatment." *American Journal of Pain Management* 5 (1995): 62–66.

Wiesel, S. W., et al. "A study of computer-assisted tomography 1. The incidence of positive CAT scans in an asymptomatic group of patients." *Spine* 9 (1984): 549–551.

Wilberger, J. E., Jr., and Pang, D. "Syndrome of the incidental herniated lumbar disc." *Journal of Neurosurgery* 59 (1983): 137–141.

Witt, I., Vestergaard, A., and Rosenklint, A. "A comparative analysis of the lumbar spine in patients with and without lumbar pain." *Spine* 9 (1984): 298–300.

Index

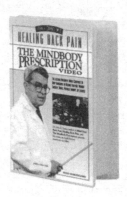